TIME TO CARE

HOW TO **LOVE** YOUR **PATIENTS** AND YOUR **JOB**

Dr ROBIN YOUNGSON

Rebelheart Publishers

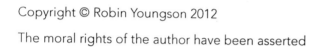

Published in New Zealand by:

Rebelheart Publishers
PO Box 63, Raglan 3265, New Zealand

Email: sales@time-to-care.com
Phone: 00 64 21 660 344

E-book editions available for download from www.time-to-care.com

Book design and cover: Emotive Design (www.emotivedesign.co.nz)

ISBN 978 1475237849

Praise for TIME TO CARE

At the critical interface between patient and health professionals TIME TO CARE offers some extremely constructive ways of salvaging care in current frenetic health service environments.
Professor Jenny Carryer, Executive Director,
New Zealand College of Nurses.

A magnificent achievement - precisely what is required in healthcare worldwide. I particularly like the fact that it presents the case for both sides: patients and staff.

TIME TO CARE is a practical manual in how healthcare professionals can give life to the value of compassion in their daily practice. A well-presented resource, which will become dog-eared and worn with use over time.

If you only read one book about healthcare in your lifetime, whether you are a patient or a professional, let this be the book. It will make a real difference to the outcome you personally experience.

One of the great strengths of the book is the very strong, compelling, evidence base to support the theory. Every medical student should be presented with a copy of this book on their first day in medical school.
Michael Brophy, Council Member,
Irish Society for Quality & Safety in Healthcare.

This book is a gem! Robin has provided the reader with a practical plan to move irrevocably from 'no-time-to-care' to 'time to care'. He's done so with humour, insight, knowledge and compassion.

TIME TO CARE is a fabulous book that provides the blue print for a model of true health care that serves not only the patients but also the good-hearted health professionals who dedicate their lives in their service.
Petrea King, Founder and CEO, Quest for Life Foundation.
Author of "Your Life Matters"

Praise for TIME TO CARE

Here is a wonderful gift from one of the pioneers of compassionate care in our health services. As the search for competitive edge drives us to do more for less until we are doing practically everything with nothing, this is a book of great wisdom and scholarship on the dangers, shortsightedness and callousness of this approach.

Well researched, beautifully written and deeply inspiring this is one book I would recommend all clinicians to read at the beginning of their careers and constantly revisit many times throughout.

Professor Paul Gilbert, OBE.
Author of "The Compassionate Mind"

I really like the book. TIME TO CARE has a very positive appeal, and it covers the topic right from the deeply personal aspects of self-renewal through to organizational aspects of culture change.

I particularly liked how the book paints a very realistic picture of what it has meant to work in the system and how it needs to be changed. There is great power in the anecdotes that will ring true with both health professionals and patients. Issues like lack of purpose, worth and meaning in the workplace are really important to address.

People feel so disconnected, so disenfranchised.... practical ways to counter these blights in the system are hugely important.

TIME TO CARE offers the choice of personal renewal, many practical ways to embody change in both individuals and organizations, and a real sense of hope for a brighter future. TIME TO CARE shows us where the light switch is. All we have to do is act.

TIME TO CARE is very simply written and will definitely appeal to both health professionals and the public. It should be an essential text in the medical student curriculum.

John Kearsley, Professor of Medicine (Conjoint),
at the University of NSW and University of Wollongong.

ABOUT THE AUTHOR

HOW TO LOVE YOUR PATIENTS AND YOUR JOB

An unassuming over-achiever, Robin Youngson was born in the UK in 1955.

An Army brat, he followed his family to postings throughout the British Empire before experiencing the horrors of institutional life in an English boarding school.

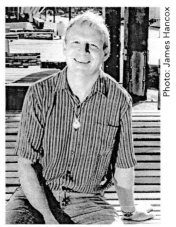

Dr Robin Youngson

In 1977 he graduated from Cambridge University with a degree in engineering, and worked for three years in the highly hazardous field of oil exploration to pay his way through medical school.

As a practicing anesthesiologist, Youngson has for years been a lone voice on the international speaking circuit for compassionate, whole patient care.

He is the founder of the international HEARTS in HEALTHCARE movement launched in 2012.

*DEDICATED TO ALL THOSE
WHO FORGOT THE RULES
AND OPENED THEIR HEARTS.*

ACKNOWLEDGEMENTS

Many people have contributed their stories, research and science in the making of TIME TO CARE and I acknowledge their contribution by giving their full name in the text. Where I use just a first name, it's an indication that I may have altered identity to preserve anonymity. These wonderful human stories are an inspiration to us all.

The research quoted in TIME TO CARE is a small summary from an extensive bibliographic database. I'm grateful to the many researchers who openly shared their work and to Ying Grace Wang who collated the database of references on the science and practice of compassionate healthcare. This bibliographic database is available to others working in the field.

The inspiration for TIME TO CARE comes from individuals who have transcended great suffering and loss to emerge as outstanding leaders in the movement to re-humanize healthcare. These humble people have little idea of the impact or importance of their work. I'm sure the readers will join me in expressing deep appreciation of their contribution and admiration for their courage and tenacity.

Our clinical work environment is not especially encouraging for those who want to talk about loving our patients. I am deeply grateful to the good people at the Australasian Integrative Medicine Association (AIMA) who offered me the very first invitation to speak about compassion in healthcare, at their 2006 conference. I would never have continued my work without their continuing support and encouragement.

I was deeply touched that an international health leader of the stature of Jim Conway would set aside so many competing demands to review TIME TO CARE and write a generous and insightful foreword. I am very grateful for his support and encouragement.

Giving up a career and income as a senior medical specialist, and trying to catalyze a worldwide movement, are rather ridiculous ideas when you have invested thirty years in medical practice. Two people deserve special mention in encouraging such insanity.

Christian Dahmen, who tragically passed away at the height of his powers, inspired many people to radically change their lives and dedicate themselves to greater purpose. He became my best mentor and a dear friend. His astonishing clarity of vision led me to discover the link between re-humanizing healthcare, the wellbeing of health professionals, and the possibilities of social movements. He believed that we could change the world.

My darling wife Meredith has encouraged me, every step of the way, to follow my heart and commit to this work. It's turned into a wonderful shared adventure, as we shed security and possessions, and partner in this quest. Her devotion, wise counsel and tactful coaching have made an enormous contribution. Meredith also brought her incisive skills in reviewing the manuscript, making many improvements, and gifting us the book title.

Finally, I give thanks to Amanda Nally of Write Answers, my editor and chief cheerleader. She had the wisdom and skills to pull apart TIME TO CARE where it needed reshaping and to give lavish praise for the bits she loved. She is part of the bigger team involving Ian Thomson at Emotive Design, which has created the book design, book cover, and also the logo and branding for HEARTS in HEALTHCARE.

Robin Youngson
April 2012

FOREWORD

In my 46 years in healthcare, I have served as a clerk, manager, administrator, executive, trustee, teacher, and lifelong student. I learned the power and privilege of patient- and family-centered care, anchored in compassion, dignity, respect, information sharing, participation, and collaboration at every level of care.

My insights were the gift of courageous communities and unique experiences at the Children's Hospital in Boston, the Dana-Farber Cancer Institute, and the Institute for Healthcare Improvement. And I learned from exciting innovators at the Institute for Patient and Family Centered Care, the Schwartz Center, the Picker Institute, Planetree, and many more.

In this long journey, I was repeatedly struck that we as leaders were not putting in place systems that supported the safe, effective, and compassionate practice of our staff. No matter how good our excellent staff is, broken systems and human error result in harm to patients. The resulting frustration and devastation on staff seems overwhelming.

I've seen the exceptional power of staff support, when there is a hug and a focus on 'What happened?' and not just 'Who did it?' This leader also observed again and again the direct correlation between a good staff experience, a positive patient experience and the power of integrated practice.

Further, observing the journey with our own patients, staff, and in worldwide practice, I consistently found islands, silos, and a lack of a community.

The 'relationship' people didn't talk either with the 'empathy' crowd or the 'compassion' advocates. The 'patient-centered' fans were different than the 'family-centered' champions and neither of them was linked to the 'family caregivers'.

For initiatives focused on the staff, the patient wasn't in the picture. I knew from other areas of practice in science and leadership that we were missing the power of shared learning and crosscutting concepts.

My hope is that the global health care conversation has now finally reached a tipping point: we are beginning to talk together about the patient, public, person, caregiver, partnerships, engagement, empathy, second victims, relationships, compassion, shared decision-making, community, and more.

We can celebrate growing awareness; in many places we are seeing changing beliefs, and in a relatively small number of islands, we are seeing changing behaviors and practices. TIME TO CARE is an inspiration for the latter.

As I began reading TIME TO CARE I wanted to stop. It begins hard and graphic; it is initially focused on inhumanity, impersonal care, what isn't working and the resultant suffering, harm, and tragedy for our patients, staff, and those who care for them.

Wherever we work in healthcare, we see staff that feels there is no longer time to care. And when we lose the privilege of serving our patients with compassion, burnout is too often the result. After 46 years I know it, I've seen it, I've felt it, but it is still distressing.

I forced myself to start reading again; Peter Senge in The Fifth Discipline taught me we have to confront the realities of practice as well as set bold aims and goals.

As I read on I got excited, really excited. I was learning things I didn't know: crosscutting concepts from positive psychology, explanatory styles, developing the habit of kindness, and the power of simple acts. The silos were being broken down.

While I'm a teacher of both 'empathy' and 'self-assessment', now I was learning new content. I was being guided to unexpected sources of insight and ideas that we can use for shared learning.

One of my favorite definitions of leadership is "Taking people to a place they didn't want to go and have them feel great that they got there."

The material on appreciative inquiry, understanding our impact on others, positive atmospheres, and mindfulness, had important new lessons for me as a leader, and I think is valuable learning for all healthcare leaders.

Those of us privileged to work in healthcare know how hard it can be on us, our patients and those who care for them. But also we also know the potential for great rewards.

Avedis Donabedian told us, "First comes love and passion, and then comes strategy and tactics." As I read TIME TO CARE I was inspired to imagine the awesome possibility and power of optimized love and passion.

The title says it all—we must find the time to care for ourselves, our colleagues, and those we serve.

In writing the book, Robin Youngson explains to health professional how they can: strengthen their hearts, choose to love both their work and their patients, gain the skills for compassionate caring, rise above institutional limitations, and join a world-wide movement to improve patient care.

The end product is a gift of crosscutting concepts and new possibilities: the imperative for change, how to do it, and why it must start with ourselves.

Jim Conway
Adjunct Faculty, Harvard School of Public Health

CONTENTS

Chapter 1

BURNOUT

In your emergency room, a patient who could be your grandmother lies untended on a gurney in the corridor. There are no beds. She's been desperately trying to attract attention but now lies mutely in soiled sheets. There was nobody to take her to the toilet.

It may not be written down anywhere but the rules for health professionals are clear: Put your head down, complete your tasks as quickly as possible, get the paperwork done, and move onto the next patient.

Yesterday you took the time to really listen to a patient, holding his hand and offering your comfort and understanding. You won't make that mistake today – not after your team members snapped at you for wasting time.

The rules are clear: Put your head down, complete your tasks as quickly as possible, get the paperwork done, and move onto the next patient

After investing hard years of training to achieve the highest qualifications – probably neglecting your family along the way – you're proud of your technical skills but now the pleasure and satisfaction of using them seems dull. The work itself is routine, day-in and day-out.

And since when did patients become so ungrateful? They neglect their health and then expect you to fix them up. Then they write complaints, or sue you when things don't turn out.

At the end of the shift you go home feeling exhausted and dispirited. Today you snapped at someone. You don't know how much longer you can keep this up.

There must be more to having a job than just earning money; it's a story more and more health workers can relate to.

Healthcare is in deep peril. The relentless progression of technological medicine, the focus on disease rather than wellbeing, the rapidly escalating costs, and the corruption of healthcare by profit making and greed are taking us fast to a crisis point. In this mad scramble, the human aspects of caring, compassion and healing are being lost.

Fatigue, depression, stress and burnout are reaching epidemic proportions in the health workforce internationally. And, as health workers become more stressed, bullying and abuse do further harm to working relationships and patient care.

The term "disruptive behavior" has debuted in medical journals in recent years [1]. It's the euphemism for toddler-style tantrums conducted by medical professionals – its hallmarks include yelling, throwing objects and slamming doors. Less flamboyant but equally damaging are weapons like sarcasm and derision.

Not the job we signed up for

Jill Maben is a researcher in London. Her fears about the state of the nursing profession were realized in a longitudinal study which showed how the ideals and values of nursing students clashed with the harsh reality of work in the British National Health Service [2].

Newly qualified nurses were exposed to a set of covert rules they were expected to adhere to, but these rules were the antithesis of their values and ideals. These four 'rules' were particularly prevalent in practice environments categorised as challenging and poor.

Rule 1: Hurried physical care prevails to the detriment of psychological care

Rule 2: No shirking! (with a need to be seen doing a fair share of the physical and 'dirty work')

Rule 3: Don't get involved with patients (keep an emotional distance at all times)

Rule 4: Fit in and don't rock the boat (don't try and introduce changes to practice)

Maben found within two years of graduation most nurses were compromised or crushed idealists. Professionally frustrated, they had a high degree of burnout leading to disillusionment, job hopping, and sometimes leaving the profession altogether.

Doctors fare no better. The Physicians' Foundation 2008 survey of 12,000 physicians in the USA painted a grim picture that could have drastic implications for the nation's healthcare [3].

The report found:

- 78% of physicians found medicine either "no longer rewarding" or "less rewarding"
- 63% of physicians said they did not always have enough time to properly treat all their patients
- 60% of doctors would not recommend medicine as a career
- 49% of physicians – more than 150,000 doctors nationwide – said that over the next three years they planned to either reduce their patient numbers or stop practicing
- 42% of physicians rated the professional morale of their colleagues as "poor" or "very low"
- Just 6% of physicians described the professional morale of their colleagues as "positive"

The chronic stress and disillusionment take their toll on staff relationships. In a survey of 50 Veterans Health Administration (VHA) community hospitals across the United States, 86% of nurses and 49% of doctors reported witnessing senior staff tantrums, which were detrimental not only to workplace relationships but ultimately to patient care [4].

Most VHA respondents believed the breakdown in communication led to medical errors, which impacted on patient safety – and sometimes even patient mortality.

Our healthcare systems are themselves causing so much unnecessary pain and suffering. Each day, our attitudes and actions are undoing much of the hard work we commit to the care of patients.

The most heart-rending accounts of that suffering come from health professionals who suddenly find themselves in the role of patients, feeling scared and vulnerable.

When health workers become patients

George Sweet, a retired psychotherapist and author in New Zealand, developed transverse myelitis, an acute inflammation of spinal nerves. Sweet described his personal experience of the hospital ward rounds [5]:

"When I first arrived in hospital I inadvertently created havoc by being honest. I had suddenly lost the use of my legs. When the ward round arrived they asked 'How are you feeling today?' I answered quite accurately: 'Very frightened, and deeply sad.' Somehow however, my answer seemed inappropriate; the team staggered cognitively, then recovered by asking about symptoms: 'Are the feet any better?' I felt dismissed, unheard. Abandoned is not too strong a word.

"I was in hospital for several months, but it took me about nine weeks to get a focus on the vagueness and dissatisfaction that these rounds produced in me. I found them to be constantly impersonal; this was exacerbated by doctors talking not with me, but amongst themselves in response to my statements. Out of anxiety I often gave quick, partial, or even unhelpful answers to questions. I did not feel that I, George, was of the slightest importance to the round. The pathology was very important. I was overwhelmed by the numbers of people who had little desire to know George or invite him to participate in his own treatment.

"Rounds usually started with a short 'How are you this morning?' I quickly learned that the correct answer was 'OK' or 'Good'. At worst, the focus seemed to be on getting an assurance that the patient was OK (which meant the round could move on), or, the patient had a problem so medications needed changing (then the round could move on). On questioning other patients, I found that 'OK' or 'Good' were also their preferred responses to the ward round style of consulting."

From my perspective as a hospital specialist, this brief account accurately portrays what I have witnessed in ward rounds in every hospital in my working life. This impersonal care is not an exception – it's the rule.

The person in the patient is quickly dissolved in the role of a patient.

Our style of medicine focuses on the disease, and standardized treatment of the pathology, not on the person with the illness. Moreover, the respective roles of practitioner and patient create a huge power imbalance.

It is much easier for patients to answer 'OK' or 'Good' in response to questions than to admit deep concerns or ask questions.

We now know this style of caring, adopted by so many health professionals, has serious consequences not only for the patient but also for the health professional.

Why we need to treat the whole person

There's growing scientific evidence of the powerful impact of emotional and psychological factors on the wellbeing and survival of our patients. For instance, in major causes of death like heart disease, the difference in death rates between pessimists and optimists is about as big as the difference between smokers and non-smokers [6].

Maybe you're a highly skilled surgeon doubting what relevance all this 'touchy, feely' stuff has to your surgical outcomes. Think again. There is conclusive evidence that if your patients are stressed, their healing will be delayed and they are at higher risk of wound infections and cancer recurrence [7,8].

Humans have extraordinary innate powers of healing. Every doctor knows patients who completely defy expectations and continue to flourish in good health when they should be dying of incurable cancer.

So, whenever we treat patients impersonally, as 'the breast lump on ward six', we fail to tap into a powerful mechanism for healing that's at least as effective as many of our medications.

This detached, impersonal style of caring is also at the heart of so much misery among health professionals. When patients feel a lack of caring, they quickly lose trust, they are dissatisfied, they feel as if you aren't listening, and they will tend to escalate their demands or withdraw. The joy of caring becomes tarnished.

And health professions tend to be their own worst critics.

The difference in death rates between and pessimists and optimists is about as big as the difference between smokers and non-smokers

As working conditions deteriorate and patient care is compromised, health workers who are heading for burnout suffer most from high levels of self-criticism and shame. It's a nasty vicious cycle, leading to depression and physical health problems.

Unhappy health professionals contaminate those around them. Bad moods are contagious. People in stressed work environments lose both patience and generosity. People snap at each other. A longitudinal study of sickness absenteeism among hospital physicians showed poor teamwork was the most powerful determinant, even greater than work overload [9].

And what happens when we run out of treatment options? Maybe the patient has chronic disease that we can't fix or cure. Worse still, incurable cancer. How do you feel when you have to tell the patient, 'I'm sorry, there's nothing more we can do'? What does that do for your sense of professional competence, your self-esteem?

Professor Keiran Sweeney was an inspirational GP and renowned medical educator in London. He died on Christmas Eve 2009, diagnosed with mesothelioma, a malignancy of the pleural lining of the lung. In a moving paper published before his death, he described his experience of learning the fateful diagnosis [10].

"The biopsy was carried out competently by a surgical team who all looked disturbingly downcast after the procedure. None could address my increasing anxiety, except perhaps the most junior member of the team, who, I sense in retrospect, did not feel he had either the authority or life experience to discuss the diagnosis. The specialist nurse came to show my wife and me how to drain the pleural catheter, which was left in to promote a pleurodesis.

"If there was anything I wanted to know about mesothelioma, he said, with the best of intentions, he had lots of information available. The physical shock of his throwaway remark fractionally preceded its violent emotional impact, but smiling blandly, I went down for a check radiograph, having been invited to do so by the nurse on duty thus: 'Could you get this young man to go down for a chest film when you're finished?' My guess is that the nurse was about 22 years old...

"While I was having the check film, my wife asked the specialist cancer nurse why everyone was so downcast. At that point, everyone around knew I had a mesothelioma, except me.

"I learnt about it by reading the discharge summary over a glass of sauvignon blanc with lunch at home: malignant mesothelioma. 'Patient is aware of the diagnosis,' said the discharge summary.

"The next 48 hours are spent talking to our four beautiful kids, aged mid-teens to early 20s, whose joyous careers are currently sprinkled through school, part time jobs, and university. I can't really convey in words the catastrophic hurt my news has inflicted on them...

"We embrace. They weep. I weep for them, for fear for myself, and for the unthinkable horror that they will continue to inhabit the world in which I will play no part. Like my wife, they are brave, selfless, and compassionate."

Sweeney went on to describe the devastating emotional impact of dealing with health professionals who were unable to acknowledge the seriousness of his illness or offer any kind of emotional support.

Sweeney's story gives insight into how much difficulty health professionals face when their treatment is directed only at the disease, or the physical symptoms of the patient. When they lack the confidence, skills, and psychological resilience to offer emotional support and understanding to a patient, they are left with a terrible failure of professional purpose.

I believe every one of Sweeney's many doctors and nurses was a caring human being, who will have suffered greatly knowing the impact of their words while feeling unable to offer comfort or hope.

But, as a health professional, if you can sit alongside patients and witness their courage, resilience, hope and forgiveness – in the face of life-threatening illness – then you feel humbled and privileged. It's a shared journey that can bring deep meaning to your work.

What happened to compassion?

Why are these practices of compassionate caring resisted so much within professional and institutional cultures? And on a personal level, what's to stop health workers from bringing their hearts to work and making an emotional connection with patients? According to the research the answers are universal:

- The sheer pace of work and multiple competing demands
- Peer pressure
- The perceived need for objectivity and clear judgment
- The de-humanizing effect of much medical technology
- Institutional rules and policies

As health professionals we are deeply immersed in a culture, which unconsciously shapes our beliefs and behaviors. These influences so powerfully inhibit compassionate, whole person care that I call them the 'tyrannies' of the system – the unconscious norms, practices, habits and beliefs we acquire in training and practice.

We seldom talk about psychological and emotional vulnerability and yet those working in healthcare witness terrible sights: horrifying injuries and mutilations (some of them in the results of treatment); disease-ridden bodies; pain and suffering; and deaths of patients who remind us of loved ones.

We're taught that the cost of emotional involvement is too high: we'd have to come to terms with our own vulnerability, brokenness, and potential mortality. How many health workers are comfortable talking with a patient about death and dying?

The first study into emotional vulnerability of health professionals was published more than fifty years ago. The classic paper is Isabel Menzies writing, A Case-Study in the Functioning of Social Systems as a Defence against Anxiety. A Report on a Study of the Nursing Service of a General Hospital [11].

Menzies' nurses were in constant contact with people who were physically ill or injured, often seriously. The recovery of patients was not certain and would not always be complete.

We seldom talk about psychological and emotional vulnerability

Nursing patients with incurable diseases was one of the nurse's most distressing tasks. Nurses were confronted with the threat and reality of suffering and death, their work involved carrying out tasks which, by ordinary standards, were distasteful, disgusting, and frightening.

Menzies reported that the nurses intimate physical contact with patients aroused strong and mixed feelings. Emotions of pity, compassion, love, guilt, anxiety warred with those of hatred and resentment which were all aroused by patients. Such strong feelings often had their root in envy of their patients for the care being lavished on them.

Menzies documented that the nurses' coping strategies reduced anxiety by de-personalizing both themselves and the patients. The strategies included:

- A 'task-list' care system, absolving nurses from the anxiety of decision-making
- Talking of patients, not by name but by disease, the pneumonia in bed 15
- Nursing uniforms becoming a symbol of behavioral uniformity; one nurse being perfectly inter-changeable with another. There is no room for the person of the nurse
- Detachment and denial of feeling. A 'good' nurse doesn't mind being moved from one job to another

Recent reports illustrate that modern day medical students have equally challenging experiences in their early clinical attachments.

Harvard Medical student Neal Chatterjee wrote [12, 13]:

"There's nothing particularly natural about the hospital – ever-lit hallways, the cacophony of overhead pages, near-constant beeps and buzzes, the stale smell of hospital linens.

This unnaturalness was strikingly apparent to me when I arrived as a third-year medical student – freshly shaven, nervous, absorbent – for the first day of my surgical clerkship.

As I joined my team, my resident was describing a recent patient: "He arrived with a little twinge of abdominal pain ... and he left with a CABG, cecectomy, and two chest tubes!"

This remark was apparently funny, as I surmised from the ensuing laughter. And the resident sharing the anecdote – slouched in his chair, legs crossed and coffee in hand – seemed oddly... comfortable.

As the year – known at Harvard Medical School as the Principal Clinical Experience – proceeded, the blare of announcements dulled to a low roar, the beeps and buzzes seemed increasingly distant, and the stale smell of hospital linens became all too familiar.

Occasionally, however, there were moments that evoked a twinge of my old discomfort, some inchoate sense that what had just transpired mattered more deeply than I recognized at the time. These moments were often lost amidst morning vital signs, our next admission, or the differential diagnosis for chest pain.

At the end of the year, we were asked to reflect, in writing, on our first year in the hospital. What eventually filled my computer screen had nothing to do with vital signs or chest pain. I began to write, "I have seen a 24-hour-old child die. I saw that same child at 12 hours and had the audacity to tell her parents that she was beautiful and healthy. Apparently, at the sight of his child — blue, limp, quiet — her father vomited on the spot." I say apparently because I was at home, sleeping under my own covers, when she coded.

I have seen entirely too many people naked. I have seen 350 pounds of flesh, dead: dried red blood streaked across nude adipose, gauze, and useless EKG paper strips. I have met someone for the second time and seen them anesthetized, splayed, and filleted across an OR table within 10 minutes.

I have delivered a baby. Alone. I have sawed off a man's leg and dropped it into a metal bucket. I have seen three patients die from cancer in one night."

The remarkable thing is that *any* health professional survives the process of training and early professional experience without becoming de-humanized. Yet some health workers are like angels, they shine in their workplace, creating oases of calm, caring and compassion.

What unique emotional and psychological strengths allow them to resist the de-humanizing influences?

Maintaining our humanity

Pioneers in the new and rapidly expanding field of Positive Psychology are studying these questions about resilience, strengths and wellbeing. For too long we have focused on mental problems like anxiety and depression, say leaders like Martin Seligman [13, 14]. We need to understand what it means to be healthy, happy and resilient. What are the psychological strengths that allow people to flourish in the face of severe adversity?

People have a great tendency to believe that differences in behavior are the result of inborn personality traits. It seems that some people are just naturally happy, carefree and resilient.

Actually these traits can be quickly learned and developed. Furthermore, instead of being perpetual victims of the world around us, we can learn to re-make our environment to create a very different life experience.

When I began this long journey of learning fifteen years ago I would have scoffed at the very concept. At the time I was an anesthesiologist doing highly specialized medicine in a big teaching hospital. My source of professional identity and self-esteem was technical expertise. While I cared about my patients, I knew little about compassionate caring.

Three things changed my mind. First the great weight of scientific evidence in related fields: the links between psychological, emotional and physical heath; the neuroscience of interpersonal connection and how profoundly we influence one-another; and the rapidly expanding science of Positive Psychology.

Second, was the gradual transformation in my own experience as I began to learn the attitudes and skills of compassionate caring. My clinical work has never been more joyful, satisfying and privileged. Jobs that used to be a chore, now give me great pleasure.

The final factor was the many stories I heard of other health professionals turning their lives around.

My email InBox has become a treasure of moving stories that begin with phrases like, "Robin, you saved my life…"

Anyone who studies evidence-based practice knows of the long lag between publication of clinical trials and adoption of that knowledge into practice. For instance, fibrinolytic therapy ("clot-busting" drugs) given within an hour of an acute heart attack can reduce mortality by up to 48% [15].

Although there was compelling scientific evidence of this benefit by the mid-1980's, the practice didn't take off until the 1990's; well into the 2000's many patients still missed out.

It's the same with evidence regarding compassionate, whole-person care and the nature of the profound interconnection between human beings: the knowledge and practice has lagged far behind the evidence.

The new field of positive psychology

The explosion of knowledge in positive psychology in the last decade is beginning to revolutionize our approach to health and wellbeing. Long-regarded practices like clinical detachment must now be re-examined in the light of modern neuroscience and our new knowledge of perception, consciousness and reality.

Prior to the millennium, almost the entire focus of psychology and psychiatry was on deficits and defects in mental health, like anxiety disorders and depression. Health was perceived as the *absence* of disease, rather than a positive flourishing of physical, emotional, mental and spiritual wellbeing.

The 'bible' for mental health practitioners is a complex classification of mental disorders called the DSM-IV. The *Diagnostic and Statistical Manual of Mental Disorders, 4th Edition* contains thousands of entries but in effect half the book is missing. There was no description or classification of mental and emotional strengths, positive values, or sources of resilience and wellbeing. Peterson and Seligman remedied this defect by publishing *Character Strengths and Virtues: A Handbook and Classification* in 2004 [16].

TIME TO CARE draws on important new evidence from the world of positive psychology. Prominent researchers like Barbara Fredrickson, the author of the best-selling book *Positivity* teach us how we can flourish as health professionals, to become the very best version of ourselves [17].

The explosion of knowledge in positive psychology in the last decade is beginning to revolutionize our approach to health and wellbeing

Now there is also accumulating evidence of the link between positive psychology and physical health. In one of many studies quoted by Seligman, Dutch seniors with high optimism had less than quarter the risk of dying of heart attack or stroke over the next decade, compared with pessimists [14].

So it becomes clear that our focus on physical disease and bio-medicine is unbalanced. We need to pay much more attention to emotional, psychological and spiritual wellbeing and the huge importance of healing relationships.

This focus on positivity, wellness, strengths and resilience – rather than disease – is foreign to health professionals. We have been so well versed in problem identification, diagnosis, treatment and risk-management that the whole character of our thinking has been unconsciously shaped.

So this new science of positive psychology is very helpful in liberating ourselves from these unconscious influences, to become fully compassionate practitioners.

Fredrickson developed a 'broaden and build' theory, which shows how positive thinking and emotions broaden our field of perception, increase creativity, and enhance our social contribution [18].

In contrast, pessimistic, unhappy thinking – focusing on problems and risks – narrows our creativity and gets us stuck in a deep rut, rehearsing our negative thoughts again and again. Did you ever have a bad day and find yourself making lists of all the things that have gone wrong already? You are priming yourself for more disasters!

This book also draws on ancient wisdom from Eastern philosophies.

Just as critical thinking styles can limit our repertoire of responses, many other unhelpful Western assumptions, frameworks and models handicap our approach to health and welfare. In the Western world, for instance, there's huge emphasis on self-esteem as a source of wellbeing. Recent research suggests that self-compassion is a far more stable foundation for happiness [19].

Our Western heroes tend to be men and women of action, rather than those with mindful consciousness and subtle influence. Compassion lies at the heart of Buddhist practice and philosophy. Taoist philosophy offers many counterintuitive ideas about leadership and influence that help us serve others more effectively.

In a remarkable coming together of ancient and modern, neuroscientists are starting to confirm many of the beliefs of Buddhist philosophy, which are based on more than two thousand years of meditation and internal study of the workings of the human mind.

These new findings from neuroscience dramatically challenge some of the core assumptions of Western scientific thinking, particularly separation of feelings and thoughts.

The dangers of clinical detachment

It may be that "clinical detachment" is a Western delusion – certainly as a concept it's deeply harmful to patient care and to the emotional wellbeing of health professionals. In contrast to a widely held belief, research shows that the doctors who are most empathetic, those who make the strongest emotional connections with their patients, actually have the lowest risk of burn-out [20, 21].

One paper reported that those trauma therapists with "exquisite empathy" defined as being highly present, sensitively attuned, well-boundaried, with heartfelt empathic engagement, were invigorated rather than depleted by their intimate professional connections with traumatized clients and thus protected against compassion fatigue and burnout [22].

It seems clinical detachment, as a psychological defense mechanism, is flawed.

In my experience, the desire for compassionate practice is never buried deep. Most health workers come into their professions with high ideals of whole-patient, compassionate care. Although our systems of healthcare often don't encourage and nurture compassion and caring, there are simple steps health workers can take that quickly lead you to a point of greater flourishing.

When we begin to shift our attitudes and beliefs, the system begins to take on a more malleable form and we find powerful ways to shape the world around us. As Gandhi said, you need to become the change you want to see.

Those who have adopted the latest developments in neuroscience and positive psychology are demonstrating that spending time actually saves time – even in the busiest and most demanding medical environments.

Doctors who make more time for caring, learn to love even their 'difficult' patients. They actually become better doctors with more successful medical outcomes. And they're happier people.

Some will say, 'Get real. You just don't understand the kind of pressure we're under every day!'

It's true. Healthcare has become incredibly stressed, patients make too many demands, and the shortage of health workers makes it all worse.

Nevertheless, there are people at work who are happy every day. They rarely get stressed and they always find time to do the special little things that make a huge difference for patients.

Doctors who make more time for caring learn to love even their 'difficult' patients

How? It turns out that many of the things we unconsciously think and do when we are stressed actually waste time, create conflict, multiply the work, make us unhappy, reinforce our stress, and make our patients more demanding.

We can learn a new way of being.

Flourishing

By doing simple things differently, anyone can flourish even in the most challenging workplace.

Dr Stephen Beeson, a family doctor in California, is one of the happiest doctors I know. His patients love him too – his patient satisfaction ratings place him in the top 1% of family doctors in the USA.

Beeson has an unusual practice: he gives his personal mobile phone number to every one of his patients. 'Feel free to call me,' he says.

Insane! Who would want to do that? Doesn't he have a family life? When I tell my colleagues to give their personal phone number to patients, they think I am mad. Patients would never let them alone.

Actually, Beeson's phone hardly ever rings. And when it does, it's usually something really important. For his patients, just knowing he's there and that he cares, is enough. They'll only bother him if it's absolutely necessary.

Beeson is an outstanding physician leader, many of the clues to his happiness are found in his book, *Practicing Excellence – A Physician's Manual to Exceptional Healthcare* [23].

The secrets to being happy and fulfilled are often paradoxical. They're hidden because the results are so unexpected. Nearly everyone imagines giving a personal phone number to patients would result in continuous calls. But the opposite happens.

Most health professionals I know spend a huge amount of time and effort every day, limiting their contact with patients. It's exhausting, managing all this demand. When you learn to trust your patients better, it's such a relief to put all that effort aside.

The more barriers built between doctor and the patient, the more they will demand of you. It's as if you're not really connecting, so patients remain unsatisfied. The more you take down your barriers and defenses, the less patients will take advantage of you. And they'll do a better job of helping themselves.

At Crestwood Medical Center in Huntsville, Alabama, Chief Nursing Officer Martha Walls, also had a crazy idea.

'I know you're busy,' she told her staff in 2007, "but on top of all your usual duties I'm going to ask you to check on each of your patients every hour. We're going to call it 'Hourly Rounds'."

Walls insisted whenever a nurse entered a room they were to follow a script. They were instructed to ask the patient about the need for pain relief, the need to use the bathroom, whether changing position would make the patient more comfortable, and did they have all their possessions in easy reach. These patient needs were high on the list of top ten reasons patients press their call button.

At first the nurses didn't exactly embrace the new practice, thinking it would interfere with their other duties. They were flat-out busy already. Now, they say, they'd never go back to the old system.

Why? Things changed in surprising ways [24]. The call-bells fell silent and the nurses found their work was interrupted less frequently. An audit showed they walked nearly a mile less per shift and spent more time on direct patient care.

After hour rounding was introduced, patient care improved too. Patient falls – a major cause of accidental patient injury – declined by 58% and bedsores reduced by 39%.

Patient satisfaction scores improved, as did the reputation of the hospital. The number of patients who would definitely recommend Crestwood to their family or friends jumped from 73% to 82% since introduction of hourly rounds.

It's a paradox: if you don't have enough time to care, slow down, stop rushing, and pay more attention. Caring doesn't take any time at all, it happens in magical moments. It turns out that investing a little time up front, in the care of the patient, is one of the magical ways of making more time to care.

A subtle shift in the attitude and behavior of the doctor elicits a more positive response from the patients. As human beings, we are deeply and intuitively sensitive to the motives and attitudes of others, mostly through non-verbal clues.

Many health professionals have told me stories of a transformational patient encounter, which marked for them a day of no return.

From that moment they found themselves on a rapidly accelerating path of positive change, with increasing joy and satisfaction in their work, greater happiness, and a growing sense of positive influence in the system.

Patient satisfaction and practitioner satisfaction are closely interrelated. This positive feedback of the cared-for patient powerfully reinforces the early changes in the practitioner and builds the courage for more openness and risk-taking in the relationship.

It turns out that investing a little time up front, in the care of the patient, is one of the magical ways of making more time to care.

When the relationship between the health professional and the patient warms up in this way, the rewards for both are immediate. There's a greater bond of trust, a deepening of mutual understanding, and satisfaction with the encounter increases greatly for both parties.

Thus both practitioner and patient find themselves on an upward spiral of enhanced positivity, which I image as a double-helix, expanding and opening as it rises.

Chapter 2
KINDNESS

All through my career in medicine, even as a student, I wondered what made me so sensitive to the plight of patients suffering in hospital. These feelings set me apart from colleagues who didn't seem to have the same empathy and concern.

One day I had an appalling revelation. With it came a painful insight into the way we institutionalize the care of patients in hospital.

Age ten, I was sent to boarding school in England. My earlier schooling had suffered badly as my father, an army doctor, was posted from country to country. Now my education was secured but the price was deep loneliness.

It's hard to convey my feeling of abandonment as I was forcibly separated from my family and locked up in a ghastly institution. The depersonalization was swift: imposition of school uniform and the loss of my given name. Henceforth I was known only as Youngson.

I slept in an unheated dormitory with about twenty others and suffered the indignity of shared bathrooms. All privacy was stripped away. Each day was shaped with a rigid timetable of events, culminating in 'lights out' at 10pm.

The food was terrible, tasteless and overcooked. We eked out the meager diet with a tuckbox of treats brought from home at the beginning of term.

Our daily life was governed by arbitrary regulations with penalties for infringements. A strict hierarchy of power and privileges kept the juniors in their place. Over all loomed the menacing figures of the matron and the headmaster. Corporal punishment was the norm.

Compulsory rugby football was a source of fear.

I was bruised and mangled in the scrum and suffered the scorn of teammates when I dropped the ball. Humiliation and punishment sometimes followed in the changing rooms. I knew what it felt to be naked and defenseless.

I was bullied for many years and felt dreadfully alone. Survival instincts kicked in, equipping me with thick skin and fierce determination. Little did I know how these events would shape my life.

So decades later my tardy revelation came with a shock: The archetypal model for the institutional culture of hospitals is the English boarding school. This is why I instinctively knew suffering, loneliness, fear and powerlessness.

Within every suffering patient I witnessed in hospital I also saw a frightened and lonely little boy. The only antidote I knew was kindness.

On entering hospital, patients are depersonalized and stripped of their power and identity; they are forcibly separated from loved ones, and have to endure many humiliations. The hospital wards closely resemble boarding school dormitories and the patients' daily routine is bound by rules and restrictions.

I recall one account of a hospital rehabilitation ward where at 'lights out' at 10pm, the walking frames were removed from the patients' bedside to stop patients wandering at night. I wondered how many frail patients might be left in soiled bed linen, if they were unable to get to the toilet in the night?

Hospital culture gives a whole new meaning to corporal punishment. In both boarding schools and hospitals, pain is inflicted to 'make you better'.

One frightened little girl, begged her parents to know when she would be allowed home from hospital.
'When you're better,' replied her mother.
'But I'm a good girl!' she pleaded.

As health professionals we are so immersed in the culture of our institutions that we barely notice what happens to patients. A rude awakening occurs when we step over to the other side of the fence.

Across the divide

Six years ago, our teenage daughter Chloe crashed her car and was critically injured. She spent three months in spinal traction with a broken neck. The technical quality of care was excellent but some of her most basic human needs were neglected.

Chloe's experience has been a major motivation for me to try to strengthen humanity and compassion in healthcare [1]. Thankfully Chloe made a full recovery.

My memory of that first traumatic day is fragmented. As a clinician, I found myself in a familiar hospital setting. In my new role as the frightened parent of a seriously injured daughter, the hospital environment seemed alien and threatening.

My strongest memories of that fateful day are the small acts of kindness done by compassionate health professionals; they gave us indescribable comfort.

In my new role as the frightened parent of a seriously injured daughter, the hospital environment seemed alien and threatening

Chloe made many journeys within the hospital: from the trauma unit to the CT scanner; back to the trauma room; onwards to the operating theatre and to intensive care. During these potentially hazardous journeys, a transit nurse watched over her.

We felt so grateful for his loving care and attention. Not only did he carry all the equipment to monitor Chloe's vital signs but he also anticipated her need for pain relief. He came equipped with morphine and other drugs to relieve her distress.

But it is the memory of one act that still brings tears to my eyes. In the junction between hospital buildings there is a join in the floor. This caring nurse stopped Chloe's trolley and individually lifted each wheel over the join to prevent her broken neck from being jolted.

It is hard to express how profoundly vulnerable and fearful one feels for a loved one in mortal danger but these acts of exquisite kindness are the things that make you feel safe.

As parents of a seriously injured teenager, we felt very lost in the strange hospital environment. This wonderful nurse took us by the hand and led us to the places we needed to be.

In the months that followed, on bad days when Chloe was suffering the most, this nurse would magically appear in her room to offer comfort. Nobody called. He just intuitively sensed when his presence was needed.

The gift of kindness

I believe that all health professionals start their training with a deep desire to provide compassionate, whole-person care to the patients and families they expect to meet, and am sure the same is true of our healthcare administrators and leaders. Even when they take actions that seem to strike at the heart of caring, they wish it could be different.

But our health professions, institutions and workplaces have evolved in ways that erode, undermine and even punish acts of caring. Many say, 'we don't have permission to care', such is the unrelenting pace of work, the focus on tasks and institutional norms of behavior.

These problems seem very vivid and real, deeply part of the system in which we are immersed. There is a sense of helplessness among health professionals and health managers. People working in healthcare feel beleaguered, all at sea, helplessly tossed by the elements.

But a much more positive viewpoint is possible.

Individuals can rediscover personal power and find ways to address these deep problems from a fundamentally different perspective, finding liberation from a tyranny of unhelpful teachings, beliefs and institutional practices.

By bringing your whole person to work – not only your professional knowledge, skills and experience but also your heart, mind and spirit – you'll discover new sources of resilience, power and influence.

Compassion is portrayed in the smallest acts. Health professionals who say they don't have time to care will find they can transform their experience by focusing on the smallest things.

Kindness is a habit, which comes quickly with practice, and you can start with your own family. Why not set your alarm clock five minutes early and do a little something for your spouse or partner before you leave for the day?

In today's stressed and over-busy healthcare environment, I meet many health professionals who deeply resent having to stay late after the end of a shift. They feel manipulated and coerced and take their bad feelings home.

Compassion is portrayed in the smallest acts But when you freely choose to give your time, for a thoughtful act of compassionate caring, you go home full of good feelings. Moreover, it gives you a satisfying sense of freeing yourself from the tyranny of workplace demands, of being a free agent.

Out in the community I heard a lovely story about a junior doctor at my hospital. A patient with a rare neurological condition was baffling the doctors. Her speech was slurred and none of the hospital staff could understand what she was saying.

Sam, the junior doctor on the ward, gave up time to sit with this patient and began to piece together her story. This new information revealed a crucial clue to her diagnosis, which required tests at another hospital for confirmation.

The ambulance arrived just after the end of Sam's shift. Knowing his patient would be fearful traveling to another hospital, and unable to make herself understood, Sam volunteered to travel with his patient in the ambulance and to act as her ambassador.

The patients' family was so impressed with this act of kindness, they told the story to many friends, who passed it on to others. I heard the story third-hand, from someone who had no idea I worked at the hospital.

You may be thinking, 'this is a lovely story but I could never do that in my frantic workplace'. Indeed, when I have polled health professionals about the barriers to compassionate and humane patient care, the commonest answer is, 'There's no time to care.'

Again, the paradoxical answer is that compassionate caring saves time, in many unexpected ways. In the meantime you can find many opportunities to show compassionate caring and kindness while simultaneously being busy with clinical tasks.

A place to start is to remember your good manners. A recent article in a prestigious medical journal argued that true patient-centered care was such a distant reality, we should at least attempt Etiquette-Based Medicine[2]. It's author M W Kahn suggests doctors observe six simple rules:

- Ask permission to enter the room; wait for an answer
- Introduce yourself, showing ID badge
- Shake hands
- Sit down. Smile if appropriate
- Briefly explain your role on the team
- Ask the patient how he or she is feeling about being in the hospital

On most of the hospital ward rounds I've seen, the average score on this list would be about two out of six items. Good manners go a long way.

Inova Health System in northern Virginia is a not-for-profit, integrated health care system serving a population of almost two million people. Inova received a four-year, $685,000 award from the Department of Health and Human Services so that a human caring model could be integrated into professional nursing practice across four hospitals[3].

They identified a number of specific behaviors that constitute caring:

- attentive listening
- making eye contact
- touching
- offering verbal reassurance
- being physically and mindfully present
- centering on the patient
- being emotionally open and available
- taking cultural differences into consideration

Listening, providing information, encouraging expressions of concern, and helping patients cope with difficult situations are all behaviors and activities that can be performed simultaneously with physical caring – they take no time. At Inova some of the necessary tasks were turned into meaningful rituals.

For instance, nurses transformed the time spent hand washing into a ritual of thanks for having the ability and privilege to care for each patient. For many the hand washing task became a time to reflect on closure and completion of the human caring experience between patient encounters.

Listening, providing information, encouraging expressions of concern, and helping patients cope

Many other changes occurred at Inova Health System, including a relentless focus on improving work processes and freeing up time to care. The impact on patient satisfaction was remarkable.

At Mount Vernon hospital, the percentage of patients scoring excellent on their patient satisfaction rose from 20.4% to 98.7%. At Alexandria Hospital, excellent ratings rose from 9.9% to 89.9%.

Nurse satisfaction score improved too. The workplace that facilitates compassionate patient care is a great place to work.

Body language

One of the markers of compassionate caring is a warm smile. But what does that constitute, exactly?

Paul Ekman is a world authority on facial expression. He trains security forces how to detect people who are lying or concealing something and his work has inspired several popular TV drama series.

In writing about the characteristics of the human smile, Ekman draws a distinction first made by a French neurologist more than a hundred years ago. Duchenne noted that there was more than one way to smile but only one type of smile accompanied positive emotions – the so-called Duchenne Smile [4].

In the genuine Duchenne Smile, the lifting of the corners of the mouth is simultaneously accompanied by contraction of the skin above and below the eyeball. When people 'smile with their eyes' we perceive them as more sincere, honest, friendly and approachable.

Most of us can instantly spot an insincere smile. When you are feeling vulnerable, the quality of smile on a nurse or doctor's face makes an enormous difference to how you feel. Are you going to experience detached, impersonal care or is this a health professional who really cares about you and anticipates the pleasure of serving you?

Very few people can fake a Duchenne smile – it encompasses an involuntary and smoothly synchronized action of facial muscles, which are coordinated in a different part of the brain than the circuits that control voluntary facial movements.

Conveying genuine warmth towards patients means you must take pleasure in the activity. Small acts of kindness and choosing to give your time are a great way to practice the genuine smile.

And beware the fake smile – it may be damaging to your health. In a study of patients with coronary heart disease, anger expressions and non-enjoyment smiles were correlated with silent myocardial ischaemia and impairment of heart function [5].

The Duchenne smile has other interesting correlations. Women who flashed a Duchenne smile in their yearbook photos as freshmen have more marital satisfaction twenty-five years later [6].

Also, when subjects are asked to give a genuine warm smile, left sided parts of the brain associated with positive emotions and approach motivation are activated. Not only does feeling good make you smile but smiling makes you feel better and strengthens pro-social behavior.

So please take care with the thoughts and feelings you bring to each patient encounter. To bring warmth and a genuine smile into the room, you may need to dispel vexed thoughts and a bad mood.

At Inova, nurses hung motivational signs over each sink and on the doors of patients' rooms to help them focus on being intentional in their work before each patient interaction [3].

Each nurse stopped before entering the room, to pause, read the message of hope and healing, and become centered on the patient encounter.

While many behaviors are consistently rated as caring or compassionate, patients may interpret the same action in strongly positive or negative ways, depending on context. Practitioners need to be acutely sensitive to the patient's perspective and pay attention to non-verbal cues in their responses.

One study explored thirteen caring behaviors with a focus group of patients [7]. A doctor empathically asked a patient diagnosed with cancer: "Is there somebody you can call or talk to?"

Some respondent cited this as an example of a very caring behaviour. Others had the opposite reaction: "That impressed me as not caring – like, don't talk to me about it, don't you have anybody in the family you can talk to?"

This unintended result hints that not all health professionals are good at judging their own skills in empathy and non-verbal communication. Some may unconsciously signal to the patient, through body language, tone of voice, or a false smile that the question 'Is there somebody you can call or talk to?' is a clear instruction to find support elsewhere.

In fact a systematic review of test of empathy in medicine showed there was quite poor correlation between physicians' self-rated empathy and the rating given by their patients [8].

The hallmarks of empathic kindness

The review suggested that the only well-validated measure of empathy using patient feedback is an instrument called CARE, The Consultation and Relational Empathy measure [9]. The ten measures in the questionnaire, rated by patients on a scale from poor to excellent, serve as a great guide to empathic practice:

1. Making you feel at ease (being friendly and warm towards you, treating you with respect; not cold or abrupt)

2. Letting you tell your story (giving you time to fully describe your illness in your own words; not interrupting or diverting you)

3. Really listening (paying close attention to what is said; not looking at notes or computer as you talked)

4. Being interested in you as a whole person (asking/knowing relevant details about your life, your situation; not treating you as "just a number")

5. Fully understanding your concerns (communicating that they had accurately understood your concerns; not overlooking or dismissing anything)

6. Showing care and compassion (seeming genuinely concerned, connecting on a human level; not indifferent or "detached")

7. Being positive (having a positive approach and a positive attitude; being honest but not negative about your problems)

8. Explaining things clearly (fully answering your questions, explaining clearly, giving you adequate information; not being vague)

9. Helping you to take control (exploring with you what you can do to improve your health yourself; encouraging rather than "lecturing" you)

10. Making a plan of action with you (discussing the options, involving you in decisions as much as you want to be involved; not ignoring your views)

An analysis of these behaviors shows three components to empathic caring:

1. **Emotional:** Observation and feedback to the patient about their feelings

2. **Cognitive:** Understanding the patient's situation and perspective

3. **Action:** Engaging with the patient to make a collaborative plan for care [10]

Those really skilled at customer service use these three components to quickly become the best friend of the complaining customer. Imagine your airline flight has been over-booked and you've just missed a crucial connection. You're feeling furious and just ready to bite the head off any airline representative!

The really effective staff member at the ticketing desk immediately notices you and smiles, asking, "How can I help you?"

In response to your furious outburst, she offers no defense but simply says, "I can see you are really angry about missing your flight." You begin to feel understood and start to calm down.

She then repeats back to you her understanding of your problem, saying, "I just want to make sure I fully understand your situation." When you correct one of the details, she repeats it back to you to double check she has it right. You now feel thoroughly understood and your temper has subsided.

She then says, "This is what I'm going to do to fix your problem..."

I ask every single patient I meet, "How are you feeling?"

While they answer me I'm carefully observing their facial expression and body language for signs of emotion. I often respond with something like, 'It's natural to feel apprehensive, is there any one thing that's causing you to worry?'

A simple statement of empathy is often enough to release the tears and uncover a fear that is deeply affecting the patient. What you learn may be crucial to your care.

In my experience, patients who are the most scared are the ones least likely to tell you what is crucially important. Using empathy to build trust and uncover hidden fears is fundamental to good practice in any setting.

Body language, facial expression, and tone of voice are all important in conveying empathy. In all cultures, empathy is conveyed in this way [11]:

1. Looking at the subject
2. Orientate your body towards the subject
3. Head leaning forward
4. Touch the forearm or upper arm
5. Facial expression – oblique eyebrows, furrowed eyebrows, lower eyelid raised, slight mouth press
6. Tone of voice

Although facial expressions of emotion are universally recognized across different cultures, the facial signs described above may code only for sadness in some cultures. But empathy and compassion are universally recognized when this facial expression is combined with the body language that signals approach and engagement.

Patients instantly pick up non-verbal cues from their caregivers and experience strong emotional reactions. Even the doctor who is practiced in clinical detachment and avoiding his or her feelings about the patient may elicit a powerful emotional response in the patient.

A study of palliative care patients explored their perceptions of caring [12]. The authors said that practitioners need to invite and develop a relationship with those they are caring for, because lack of empathy and compassion can be devastating:

"I was told the bad news by the coldest woman that I ever met in my life… She was a snake to me."

"The consultant and registrar walked past about three times, the door was wide open and the consultant didn't hand wave, didn't smile, or anything."

Conversely, an empathetic response is deeply meaningful:

"The oncologist said, 'so, tell me about yourself'… I was so stunned because nobody had ever said that. . . usually you're just a melanoma or a bunch of symptoms."

"I remember getting on the phone to the doctor and crying. She said, 'I'll do what I can' then she said, 'I'm sorry, it sounds like a complete nightmare.' That was a very short sentence but it was recognition of what we were going through."

But what if I don't like my patient?

One author describes empathy as "emotional labor" in the practitioner-patient relationship, drawing an analogy with types of acting employed by stage and screen actors [13].

In the method-acting tradition, actors engage deep emotional and cognitive memories and reactions to bring their performance to life. They literally feel their parts and convey emotion naturally.

In contrast, surface acting employs a voluntary manipulation of behavior, tone of voice and facial expression and to convey the right emotions, without a corresponding emotional and cognitive underpinning.

In patient care we need to engage in emotional labor using both deep acting and surface acting. Although deep acting is preferred, practitioners may have to rely on surface acting when immediate emotional and cognitive understanding of patients is impossible.

For instance, not all patients elicit our sympathy. Some seem more deserving of our care than others. When treating patients who are unpleasant, rude, threatening, violent or grossly irresponsible it may be impossible to feel sympathy but we can still use the practice of empathy.

We can still show an appreciation of their suffering and an understanding of their situation even if our feelings are dissonant with our actions. This is surface acting, where we voluntarily suppress expressions of anger or disgust and do our best to provide good care. It carries an emotional toll.

In deep acting, we engage our hearts in our work and suffer with the patient. Compassion allows us to transmute that suffering into a positive emotion and to derive deep satisfaction from the relationship.

Over time, with the practice of compassionate caring, we steadily enhance our resources for wellbeing, resilience and self-compassion in the upwards spiral of positivity and flourishing.

Non-judgment

As we increase our stores of equanimity and loving kindness, we find ourselves judging less. With empathetic understanding, difficult patients seem to melt away. When we are called to care for those who do harm in society, we are more likely to perceive the deep suffering that drives their destructive behavior.

As we learn to ease our moral judgments, the need for surface acting declines and compassionate caring becomes easier. We less often experience the dissonance between feelings and actions and the emotional labor of caring decreases.

When we connect to our patients as real people, we learn more about their lives and find opportunities for greater understanding. One day a patient who arrived very late for a planned cesarean section disrupted my operating schedule.

My annoyance at this 'irresponsible' patient vanished when I learned she had walked for two hours, carrying her bag, to get from her home to the hospital – she had no car and no money for a bus fare. She was heavily pregnant and hadn't been allowed to eat or drink, in preparation for surgery.

Walking the TALK

Non-judgment is a hard task. It takes time and effort to hone your skills in empathy. Skills in body language don't come to all of us naturally. And we can struggle to be mindful when so many things demand our attention.

Yet there is one habit all of us can start today.

I call it Tiny Acts of Loving Kindness.

If you want to become happier in your practice, you have to 'Walk the TALK'.

Here's an example: My wife and I have recently been traveling. At all the tourist spots, we'd see couples taking photographs of the scenery with their partner in the foreground. Meredith, my wife, delights in asking, would they like her to take a photograph of the scene with both of them in it?

This kind suggestion has always been greeted with happy surprise, and often a reciprocal favor is offered. A common language is not required because the suggestion is easily made with sign language. Every time, this little act of kindness resulted in smiles and appreciation. It's really fun to do.

Researchers in positive psychology have shown there is no more powerful way to begin to increase your stores of positivity and happiness. Tiny acts of loving-kindness are the bedrock of happy and fulfilling practice. The habit of kindness will enhance and strengthen all the parts of the brain concerned with loving kindness, empathy, non-judgment and pro-social behavior.

So here are some ideas. Most of these things take just a moment. Some take a little longer but they all involve making a positive choice about how you spend your time.

1. On the drive to work, stop to let people into the queue. Give them a smile.

2. When you see someone looking lost in the hospital corridor, ask if you can help. Then take them to the place they're seeking, rather than giving directions.

3. Do something for the comfort of a patient – fetch an extra pillow or warm blanket.

4. Send an unexpected note of thanks.

5. Make sure the most junior staff get their break first.

6. Offer to walk down with the anxious patient going off the ward for a test.

7. Send a text message to let someone know you are thinking of them.

8. Greet a consulting member of staff with a smile, introduce the patient and find the notes.

9. When you find a patient in pain, attend to that first before anything else.

10. Bring fresh-baked cookies to work.

11. If a family is anxiously waiting for a loved one to finish surgery, offer to take their phone number and make the call to let them know their loved one is safe.

12. When you finish a consultation at the bedside, make sure the patient's water jug is in reach.

13. Before you leave, ask if there is anything else you can do. Say, 'I have the time'.

14. Give a donation to the charity collector.

15. When the patient is going home from the hospital, make a call to the family doctor.

16. When visiting a dependent person in the community, give them a call and ask if you can get anything from the corner shop on the way.

17. Make a new student feel welcome – introduce yourself, show interest, and teach something.

18. Give a colleague appreciative feedback – say you noticed them doing so-and-so, and how much you appreciate that.

19. Phone your patient to let them know the result of a test.

20. At the queue in the work cafeteria, let a hurried person into the queue in front of you.

21. For the patient that needed more time, go back at the end of your shift and spend some time listening.

You'll be amazed how much this simple habit lifts your mood and enhances your enjoyment at work each day. Your life partner or spouse might notice a difference too!

But how do we deal with tragedy? The reality is, healthcare can be a brutalizing environment to work in. How do we retain our humanity and compassion when witnessing overwhelming tragedy, suffering and loss?

Chapter 3

TRYING TO SURVIVE

When I had been a doctor for exactly nine days, I did my first weekend on-call. My shift started at 8am on Saturday and ended at about 6pm on Monday. In that time I had three hours' sleep.

Over the weekend, I admitted and treated only fifteen emergency patients. By usual standards, it was a small number. But six of these patients died, despite my best efforts.

Some died suddenly, of cardiac arrest following a heart attack. My entire weekend was punctuated with frantic bleeps from my pager, signaling that yet another patient had coded on coronary care.

Resuscitation was often a frantic, messy affair. Desperation, confusion and haste saw iv lines ripped out, drug ampoules dropped, and critical monitors accidentally disconnected. Cardiac massage is an unnatural act.

Most often, the attempted resuscitation was unsuccessful. The end result was shocking. I had never seen a freshly dead person before.

Going to tell the family of a patient that our efforts had been futile filled me with dread. I had no preparation for this challenging task and I felt profoundly incompetent and inadequate in dealing with these sudden, life-threatening emergencies.

More than once, my giving the news of a loved one's death was interrupted by the cardiac arrest pager. I returned shamefaced, with yet another death on my conscience, to complete the task.

One patient bled to death from a gastric ulcer. He vomited blood everywhere and had a cardiac arrest.

Another presented in coma from a massive stroke. One died of acute heart failure, desperately agitated and breathless. Among the survivors were patients with severe asthma, meningitis, emphysema, and septic shock.

During the weekend I was supervised by a resident, who at least had a few years of experience. On the Monday morning I was abandoned. The resident was on leave and my consultant was busy doing a clinic. I was completely out of my depth.

My consultant phoned me to ask if I had yet done the lumbar puncture on the patient with suspected meningitis. This terrifying procedure involved sticking a four-inch needle into the patient's spine. I had never even seen the procedure done, let alone performed it.

I worked frantically through the three days and nights, too busy to stop for meals or to sleep. The list of tasks in my notebook grew ever larger. I did my best to remain calm, to prioritize tasks, and use my meager knowledge and skills to fend off death and disaster.

When I left hospital, six of my patients were still seriously ill. I cycled home five miles, weeping helplessly. The pent up terror and grief of the nightmarish three days was finally released.

My wife sent a reasonably sane husband to work on Saturday morning and a complete wreck returned home on Monday evening. The dreadful cycle was to be repeated endlessly, 36 hours on, 12 hours off. I returned home and slept every second night.

My wife sent a reasonably sane husband to work on Saturday morning and a complete wreck returned home on Monday evening

As the years progressed, some semblance of competence began to emerge. The intense fear lessened. The inhumanity did not.

Six years later, working as a senior resident in anesthesiology one Saturday afternoon, I witnessed in quick succession the deaths of a young mother, her baby, and then a nineteen year-old motorcyclist. We are accustomed to seeing old people die. Young deaths are so much more shocking.

I was rostered on a 'long-day' fourteen-hour shift. After completing all the paper work and reporting the deaths to the Coroner's office, I had a cup of tea. In the remainder of my shift I anesthetized five more patients.

The legal requirements of informed consent include listing all the major potential complications and risks.

As I stood at the bedside of my next patient, I wondered silently if I should tell him that my last three patients all died? I decided to keep quiet.

It didn't occur to anyone in the hospital that I should be stood down, take time off work, or receive trauma counseling to deal with the emotional aftermath of such horrifying events.

A patient once confessed to me that she perceived the hospital doctors to be cold and impersonal, like robots. 'Is this me?' I thought.

Vulnerability

The defense against such emotional trauma is a suit of armor made of professional expertise and heroic doctoring. After qualifying as a doctor, it took me nine more years of training and endless exams to finally become a staff anesthesiologist in a major teaching hospital.

In our weekly departmental morbidity and mortality meetings, we swapped tales of derring-do. How, in the face of overwhelming illness or major injury, we somehow saved lives. We conspired to reassure ourselves that poor outcomes were not our fault.

While the details of technical care were turned over and dissected, the subject of our emotions, feelings, fears and vulnerabilities were off the table altogether. These are taboo subjects in the hospital medical culture.

I worked at my last hospital for eleven years. In that time, only once did I hear a senior doctor speak of personal vulnerability, openly, in front of others. He was an obstetrician and gynecologist who confessed to me in the operating room, in front of the nurses, that he hadn't felt like coming to work today.

The day before, a cesarean section had gone horribly wrong and the patient nearly bled to death. The surgical team fought for six hours to save her life, replacing her complete blood volume over and over. Eventually she stabilized enough to get her to the intensive care unit. This surgeon told me he was so traumatized by the events, he had just wanted to stay at home today, not do a list of gynecology cases.

In the last decade, that is the only time I have heard such a public confession of vulnerability from a senior hospital doctor.

Yet our failings and mistakes injure and kill patients every day. The accepted figure for the proportion of hospitalized patients, who are accidentally harmed in the course of healthcare, varies between 10% and 40% of all patients. Medical error is a leading cause of death.

This internal tension between our heroic, fearless ideal of doctoring, and the reality of so many patients that we cannot save, or we accidentally harm, is a source of tremendous emotional vulnerability.

For much of my career as a senior hospital specialist, my source of self-identity and self-esteem was technical expertise. When I couldn't save a patient or, worse still, caused accidental harm, I felt a terrible failure of professional purpose. Moreover, I didn't have the capacity for compassion and caring that might have given the patient comfort in the face of loss and suffering.

Sometimes we feel very alone in our shame. Every doctor has a case like this, where the guilt and shame burn on.

I was a new senior resident in anesthesia, rostered solo to anesthetize a patient for major vascular surgery. I'd worked in the hospital only a week and I didn't know the surgeon or the operating room staff. I didn't know where to find essential equipment and I was unfamiliar with local procedures and protocols. To make matters worse, all cases started late that day because the anesthesia department had a meeting.

When I couldn't save a patient or, worse still, caused accidental harm, I felt a terrible failure of professional purpose

My high-risk patient needed an arterial line, a central line and an epidural as part of the anesthetic management.

I struggled with every procedure, wasting time. The waiting surgeon grew impatient, then angry, and stopped talking to me.

Both the surgery and the anesthetic went badly. The patient proved to have a sicker heart than pre-op tests predicted. I couldn't control the blood pressure. The essential communication and coordination between surgeon and anesthesiologist was lost. The patient bled profusely. I struggled alone and didn't call for help. Where I had trained in the UK, asking for help was not part of the culture.

In the middle of the day, one of the senior anesthesiologists stepped into my operating room. He said, 'I noticed there was a new resident doing a major case alone so I thought I'd see if you needed help.'

He quickly realized I was in serious difficulty. He sent me out for a break and by the time I returned, he had greatly improved my patient's condition. I was deeply grateful for his empathic support and practical help. While I was glad for my patient, I felt ashamed of my failings.

My patient went to intensive care and his condition gradually worsened. Every time I was on-call, this patient appeared on the list of acute cases for the operating room. I felt like he was haunting me. I took him two more times to the operating room for treatment of complications but his condition deteriorated. He died after a month in intensive care.

I'm sure it's the worst anesthetic I have given. This patient's death hangs on my conscience. I thought I was competent to do the case but have since come to understand that I was set up to fail on that day. No doctor could have performed well in those circumstances.

Experiences like this are traumatizing for the doctor, creating fear and vulnerability. Both my patient and I were abandoned by an unsafe system – save for my kindly rescuer. The patient's relatives live with their loss, I with my shame.

Nurses face a different set of challenges, owing to their intimate connection with patients. Kathleen Galvin and Les Todres are researchers in the UK, applying humanistic frameworks in their exploration of what nursing open-heartedness means. Their paper explores the nurse's response to a series of fictional but challenging patient encounters [1].

The first vignette is a death scene:

> "The scenario is a death bed. It is not a peaceful scene. The room is brightly lit and it is a hot day outside in the garden. The young woman of 22 is fighting for air; she is angry and her young but broken body, savaged by chemotherapy, is fighting to live as it is dying. Each breath brings a rasp, a low, throated gasp which signals her determination to fight … to hold on to her rapid breathing.
>
> The nurse standing at the bedside is the same age; her task is to be present. The nurse can feel the young woman's anger, her bitter fight; she identifies with it, but she also senses that it is not her anger because she is not the other. There is a boundary between her own body and the dying body before her, but the nurse is still intensely frightened."

The authors ask, what kind of open-heartedness can bear the possibility of the other not having a good death? How does the nurse deal with an overpowering sense of futility and yet still remain present for the patient?

And how does the nurse bear the possibility "this could be me"? In the face of such distress and fear, it's easier to distance oneself and "to busy about in a professional manner, leaving the dying alone in the gravity of her situation."

The second vignette is one of humiliation:

> The scenario is fecal incontinence. A man of 45 is laid on his back in a hospital bed on an open ward with seven other patients. It is the middle of the day and meals are about to be served. He is lying in his feces and he is in pain. He cannot move and is aware of the stench of his feces and the presence of other patients.
>
> He has been like this for five minutes but he knows the nurse is on his way; he has gone to get a bowl, cloths, and water. He feels a degree of self-disgust, even self-loathing; an overpowering anxiety, a deep worry that everyone around is also extremely averse to this situation and is bearing this smell resentfully. He wants to be invisible, not noticed.

The authors explored the dual nature of the body. In the complexity of embodiment, openheartedness acknowledges both body as carnal matter and body as soulful window to the depth of a life.

The sensitive nurse will be able to maintain a respectful and intimate distance in acknowledging the shared experience of the body object being unreliable: "As you get stronger this won't happen, it is just your body saying I am really tired and sick right now."

At the same time he can empathize with the patient's humiliation, working quickly and gently to wash the patient and change the soiled linen while also acknowledging, "This won't take long... I know it's not OK."

And yet Maben's research, quoted in Chapter 1, reminds us of the reality of the working environment and the covert rules governing nursing care [2]: Hurried physical care prevails; no shirking; don't get involved with patients. The unwritten rules of the institution undermine openhearted compassion and caring.

When health professionals are abused and de-humanized by an uncaring system, how can we expect them to show compassion to their patients? There's only so much distress professionals can bear and there comes a point where emotional detachment is the only survival strategy. Why are we surprised with the high rates of burnout?

Taking off the armor

It will take time to change the professional culture in our institutions. One day we'll wrap young health professionals in a supportive environment that encourages humanity, compassion and vulnerability.

Meanwhile, there's much you can do to heal your own wounds, reduce your fear and vulnerability, and bring all of yourself to the compassionate care of patients – not just your technical expertise. The source of that healing is the love and understanding of your patients.

When you have strengthened your heart and increased your positivity and resilience, it's time to take a risk and open yourself up to your patients. For me it felt like taking off a heavy suit of armor [3].

In August 2002, a terrible accident occurred in the Maternity operating room at Waitakere Hospital, in Auckland, New Zealand [4]. A seventeen-year-old patient having a cesarean section under spinal anesthesia caught fire when the alcohol-based skin disinfectant applied to her skin was accidentally ignited.

The fire burnt unseen under the surgical drapes, searing skin that was numb and anesthetized. When the flames reached un-anesthetized skin on the upper part of her body, the patient realized that something terrible was happening. Just as she screamed in anguish, the surgical drapes melted and everyone in the operating room became aware that a major fire was burning.

The swift action of the professionals prevented the baby from being harmed. The fire was extinguished, the patient given a general anesthetic, the surgical site was re-prepped, and the baby safely delivered. The patient suffered full-thickness, third-degree burns to sixteen percent of her body surface. She required multiple skin grafts and is scarred for life.

I was the Clinical Leader of the hospital where this accident occurred. Over the next five weeks, I worked intensively with the General Manager and the Director of Nursing to manage the aftermath of this awful accident.

One of the stressful aspects of this experience for me was being interviewed on national TV news, answering the question, "Doctor, can you explain to us how you managed to set fire to one of your patients?" I was not the patient's clinician but as clinical leader of the hospital I had a compelling sense of responsibility for the safety of all of our patients.

The reason I can write about this case is that all of the details are in the public domain. Back in 2002, we were one of the first public hospitals in New Zealand to employ apology and open disclosure. We believed strongly that our moral duty was to minimize further harm to the injured patient and to help her heal and recover. Honesty and openness were essential parts of our strategy.

We employed a forensic investigator and assembled a team of enquiry comprising representatives from all the different statutory authorities.

We gathered the evidence and swiftly conducted interviews with the staff involved in the accident.

We believed strongly that our moral duty was to minimize further harm to the injured patient and to help her heal and recover. Honesty and openness were essential parts of our strategy

We pieced together the causes of the accident. We gave daily support to the injured patient, her family, and the health professionals involved in this terrible accident. The media scrutinized our every action – we were front-page news within a day of the accident.

In a series of media conferences, we shared our growing understanding of the causes of the accident. Before each meeting with the news media, we briefed the patient and her family and negotiated with them what could be revealed, and what kept confidential.

Five weeks after the accident, our final report was published [4]. Both the clinicians and the hospital were exonerated. The system failures underlying the accident were widely reported and international patient safety alerts were published – many other hospitals unknowingly faced the same risk factors.

In all of this, our patient never blamed the clinicians or the hospital. There was no letter of complaint and she chose not to sue the hospital for damages, even though we shared with her all the evidence of our failings.

When the young mother subsequently published her story in one of the weekly women's magazines, she did so on condition that the hospital not be named and no blame assigned to the health professionals. She said, "These doctors, nurses and midwives are my heroes – their swift action saved my baby and prevented further harm to me."

The health professionals present in the operating room that day were traumatized. In many hospitals in the world, they would have been instructed to avoid all contact with the patient, deny all liability, and let the lawyers handle the fallout. In all probability the impending lawsuits would have hung over them for years.

In contrast, our clinicians had the chance to heal their wounds. They maintained a therapeutic relationship with the patient and family, making frequent visits. As the patient recovered from her injuries, so the wounds in the hearts of the clinicians healed also. Her forgiveness helped them deal with their guilt and shame.

It turns out that patients don't very often expect us to be heroes. They expect us to be competent, careful, and to do our best. When we make mistakes, they want us to learn from them and to prevent this bad thing from happening to someone else.

I am humbled by the willingness of patients to forgive mistakes. It seems they value caring, compassion, humanity and sincere apology more than impersonal technical performance.

Why patients sue their doctors

When patients sue their doctors, financial compensation is rarely the primary motive. No amount of money can compensate for loss and tragedy.

But too often, hospitals and doctors take a defensive stance that denies the patient any apology, explanation, or a sense that the lessons have been learned from the error.

Dr Marie Bismark is dual qualified as both a doctor and a lawyer. Her interests led her to research the motives of patients making complaints after healthcare error, and different systems of compensation.

In a wonderful essay on the power of apology, Bismark tells the story of how friends came to lose their precious son through medical error [5].

Justin Micalizzi was a healthy 11-year-old boy who loved to play sport with his friends. One day he developed a painful, swollen ankle and fever. He was taken to the operating room for a simple procedure to incise and drain the infection. He never woke up. By the next morning he was dead.

The hospital system failed Justin's grieving parents twice: first their precious son died and then the hospital neglected to explain to them why, or even apologize for the loss of their son.

Nearly eight years later, Justin's mother – Dale Ann Micalizzi – wrote:

> "I am still waiting for, and still need that conversation. Not receiving an apology and explanation from someone caring for your child when something goes wrong is incomparable to any form of inhumanity in medicine or in society. It is simply not right.
>
> Justin was our child and we were owed an explanation and an apology. We didn't expect anyone to say, "I'm sorry I screwed up". But perhaps simply, "I am so very, very sorry that your son has died in our care. I will do everything in my power to help you and your family heal and explain to you everything that I honestly know about the event."
>
> Justin's surgeon would have been my hero if he said that to us but instead they said "these things happen in medicine" and we were expected to accept that. As a parent, I couldn't."

Patients sue because they are denied answers. They feel abandoned by their doctors. Human caring and compassion are missing. Financial compensation only serves to cheapen their losses. Money does not heal emotional wounds.

A friend in the USA fell off his ladder and broke his elbow. The injuries he sustained in the course of his hospital care compounded his suffering.

A surgeon, accidentally using the wrong jig to guide the placement of screws in the bone, drilled into my friend's arm too close to the elbow. He managed to hit the radial nerve and wrap it around the drill bit. When my friend woke up, his arm was partly paralyzed from the nerve damage, a permanent injury.

During later surgery, his elbow joint was infected with the MRSA super-bug, resulting in months of severe pain, fear of losing his arm, and the side-effects of long-term antibiotic therapy.

To add insult to injury, the hospital billing department accidentally added a zero to the cost of an implant. When my friend refused to pay, the hospital threatened to bankrupt him.

He sued for damages, not because he wanted to punish the surgeon but because he had suffered serious financial losses owing to the mistakes in care. The day he received his check, he told me, felt like the worst day of his life.

He felt like he had sold out. No amount of money would compensate for his suffering; receiving money from the insurance company didn't tell him that the surgeon cared, or had learned from his mistake. As far as the hospital was concerned, it was a 'closed claim'. My friend still waited for an apology or explanation.

But after serious medical error, it's not only the patient who is injured. Doctors can find themselves the second victim, wounded and grieving over the consequences of their actions.

Living with mistakes and failures

In 1999, Harvard anesthesiologist Dr Rick van Pelt nearly killed a fit young patient who came for ankle joint surgery. As part of the anesthetic technique, he injected local anesthetic around a nerve behind the knee, to render the foot numb and ease the pain after surgery. Unfortunately, he inadvertently injected some of the local anesthetic drug into a vein where it was carried to the heart.

The patient, Linda Kenney, suffered a severe toxic reaction and had a cardiac arrest. Initial resuscitation efforts proved futile. By great good fortune, the next-door operating room was set up and ready for open-heart surgery, complete with a primed heart-lung bypass pump. The arrested patient was rushed into the cardiac operating room, her chest opened, and her failed circulation taken over by the heart-lung machine. In a few minutes her normal heartbeat was restored and she was taken to intensive care.

Kenney went to sleep expecting ankle surgery and woke up on intensive care with a huge wound in her chest. Fortunately she survived the prolonged resuscitation without brain damage. Dr van Pelt wanted to offer sincere apology and explanation to his patient but the hospital authorities forbad him from making any contact with the patient. Over the next six months, the guilt of his error and the abandonment of his patient weighed heavily on his conscience; to the extent he wondered if he could continue his medical practice.

Eventually he decided to defy the hospital authorities and wrote a letter of sincere apology to Kenney. She rejected this advance, overwhelmed with anger at the lack of timely apology or explanation and feeling cynical about the motives of her doctor who had nearly killed her through his negligence.

The patient realized that her doctor was as wounded by this accident as she was

After more than a year of standoff, doctor and patient finally met. The anger and hostility dissolved in mutual forgiveness and support. Kenney realized that her doctor was as wounded by this accident as she was.

This courageous doctor and patient now tour the country speaking together about their experience. They set up a non-profit organization in 2002 to help doctors and patients cope with the aftermath of medical error and to promote compassion, healing and forgiveness.

The Medically Induced Trauma Support Services (MITSS) [6] exists to "To Support Healing and Restore Hope" to patients, families, and clinicians who have been affected by an adverse medical event.

A comprehensive review of the experience of doctors after medical error identifies how much doctors suffer from their mistakes [7]:

One surgeon, Atul Gawande, now renowned for his international work on surgical safety, describes his feelings after trying, and failing, to intubate a trauma victim and waiting too long to call for help.

"I felt a sense of shame like a burning ulcer. This was not guilt: guilt is what you feel when you have done something wrong. What I felt was shame: I was what was wrong."

Another doctor wrote about his experience at a rural hospital in South Africa doing his best to provide maternity care with no specialist backup. He waited too long to intervene with cesarean sections on two deliveries. Both babies died.

"At this point, I wanted to run away, to hide, to weep, to give up medicine – anything but go and tell that mother that her baby was dead."

He felt like a murderer and wanted to leave medicine, but forced himself to go back to work, all the time questioning himself, "Am I competent?"

Psychiatrist Michael Rowe witnessed the death of his own son from multiple complications after liver transplant. He interpreted the long silence from doctors after his son's death as a lack of compassion.

Rowe explains it was their perceived coldness – rather than medical error per se – which led him down the path toward legal action [8].

The most moving story, I heard from a colleague in Tasmania. Christopher Newell was both a medical school professor and an Anglican priest. Born with a severe congenital illness, Newell was not expected to survive beyond his teens. He reached his forties and I heard him speak at a conference not long before his death. He rode to the podium on an electric wheelchair and required supplementary oxygen to give him enough breath to speak.

Newell explained that he had spent about half his life in hospital. He had frequent exacerbations of his chest condition, precipitating sudden collapse. One day he would be a medical school professor with status and power. The next he'd find himself in hospital, helpless as a baby.

He had long come to accept that brokenness was part of the human condition. But the hopelessness of his condition was a threat to the feelings of competence of the nurses and doctors who treated him. They felt they had to do something to make him 'better'.

With great emotion, Christopher described one health professional who was willing to sit with him and offer "non-anxious presence". That, he said, was the most deeply therapeutic and healing moment in all his years of hospital treatment.

Fixing, helping or serving?

Rachel Naomi Remen writes of the difference between "fixing, helping, and serving" [9].

She said trying to fix patients can be a form of judgment. If someone needs fixing, it implies we think they must be broken.

While that's perfectly appropriate for someone with a broken leg, it can get in the way of treating a patient with chronic illness or disability.

Remen explains helping patients is laudable, but there is a power relationship implied in helping. The "helper" retains the knowledge, power and influence. The patients being helped tend to take a passive role, disempowered from helping themselves.

Most of my career, I tried to fix and help patients. If those are the only roles we know, we make ourselves responsible for every single life problem, dissatisfaction, and health problem in our patients' lives – because we disempower our patients. Ultimately, that is the source of the overwhelming demand faced by healthcare.

Remen said serving people was different. When people are being served, the hallmark of that relationship is that the person being served grows. When we truly serve our patients, they grow in their capacity to deal with life's problems and find the healing they need.

Remen's distinction between these three modes of treating patients solved for me a puzzling paradox. When lately I decided that I would try to respond to every concern brought by my patients, and take down all my barriers, the demand of my patient grew less, not more. How could this be?

Earlier I had discovered the power of shifting my own attitude and decided that 'difficult' patients were my own invention; the problem was the doctor, not the patient. This change in attitude miraculously dissolved all my experience of difficult patients.

I began to wonder if I could take a step further and assume that no patient makes unreasonable demands?

What would happen if I tried to respond to every concern brought by a patient?

My colleagues thought I was mad. Their daily experience is patient demand far exceeds the care resources available. We have to expend a great deal of energy managing and limiting the access of patients. We make our appointments shorter and shorter, ration care, deny access to treatments, put up costs, make patients wait, and employ numerous other strategies to conserve our limited resources.

But when I tried to make myself open to every patients' concern, the response was paradoxical. My patients' demands were reduced.

The fundamental difference is that I tried to serve the patients on their own terms. In any consultation, I did my best to first find out what was most important to the patient. I then brought my knowledge, skills, expertise and influence in the service of that concern.

I noticed that the quality of my relationship with patients changed. There was more trust and greater appreciation. My patients seemed to walk out of the consultation standing a little taller. Somehow they felt more validated, acknowledged, and understood. With that greater sense of self, they perceived that they could solve many of their own problems.

I noticed that the quality of my relationship with patients changed. There was more trust and greater appreciation

I also found that I no longer needed to be the expert all of the time. I could admit uncertainty or confusion. If I didn't have the answer I could help the patient find alternatives for treatment or care.

I enjoyed being an advocate for patients, helping them navigate their way around the complex healthcare system. I could use my influence and power on their behalf.

Sometimes I found that listening was the most important thing I did. I didn't feel compelled to offer treatment or advice. When people told me their stories, it felt like a privilege to have a front seat in their life adventures. I was amazed by the courage, resilience and humor I heard from people facing awful difficulties and life-threatening challenges.

Self-compassion and gentleness

I became a better doctor when I acknowledged my own human failings. I have my own vulnerabilities and blind spots, I make errors, and I am sometimes fearful and uncertain. When I judged myself harshly, I was also less kind to my patients. When I was more accepting of my flaws, I judged patients less.

For a long time I didn't understand non-judgment. When my life-coach suggested I try non-judgment as a life principle, I railed against the idea. I protested that my professional value lay in the exercise of judgment. Why else had I trained for so many years to become a highly qualified expert? It hadn't occurred to me that there was another form of judgment.

One of the keys to compassionate caring is self-compassion. The leading authority on self-compassion, Kristin Neff, says, "Self-compassion entails being kind and understanding toward oneself in instances of pain or failure rather than being harshly self-critical.

It's a case of perceiving one's experiences as part of the larger human experience rather than seeing them as isolating; and holding painful thoughts and feelings in mindful awareness rather than over-identifying with them." [10].

A self-compassion questionnaire included self-kindness items like:

I try to be understanding and patient towards those aspects of my personality I don't like.

I'm kind to myself when I'm experiencing suffering.

When I'm going through a very hard time, I give myself the caring and tenderness I need.

I'm tolerant of my own flaws and inadequacies.

I try to be loving towards myself when feeling emotional pain.

Descriptors on the self-judgment sub-scale include:

I can be a bit cold-hearted towards myself when I'm experiencing suffering.

I'm disapproving and judgmental about my own flaws and inadequacies.

I'm intolerant and impatient towards those aspects of my personality I don't like.

Harshly self-critical health professionals have a hard time being kind to themselves and can struggle to show compassion to their patients.

In fact stress, burnout and depression result in impaired patterns of professional conduct similar to what is seen with substance abuse [11].

This impairment may diminish productivity, lead to medical errors and compromise patient safety.

Many professionals in the Western world rely on self-esteem as a source of self-worth but that is often contingent on outcomes.

Health professionals who make mistakes suffer badly because it dents their self-esteem and sense of worth. However, self-compassion may be a more stable foundation for self-worth and wellbeing [12].

As I have let go of the compelling need to apply my technical and clinical skills and to approach my patients more humbly, I have learned to be more patient and gentle.

Two years ago I was fortunate to spend five days at the Quest for Life Foundation [13] and see the wonderful Petrea King at work. I joined a residential program with twenty others who were seeking peace, happiness and the healing of old wounds.

Many participants told horrifying stories of tragic loss, serious illness, violent abuse or other burdens that shaped their lives. I spoke of the trauma and brutalization I had experienced in my medical practice.

What I learned from King was gentleness and non-judgment in the approach to peoples' vulnerabilities.

My medical habits and expectations did not sit easily within a program that seemed so passive and so full of inactivity. The daily lunch break yawned from 1 until 3.30pm. At my hospital I usually grab a quick sandwich while working at my desk!

Each day began with an hour of relaxation and meditation. Our meals were prepared with seasonal organic food. Counseling and massage therapy were on tap. Slowly, day-by-day, the peace of the place dripped into you.

King made no attempt to overcome resistance. In her infinitely gentle, compassionate and wise way, she simply bore witness to suffering. She invited participants to let go of past events and to stop fretting about the future. She called us all to "come to our senses" – literally to connect to the present moment through mindfulness and noticing our rich sensory experience.

As the days passed, I began despair that some of the participants would ever climb out of their anger, depression, anxiety, or self-loathing. One lady had spent four days curled up on the floor in a fetal position, hugging cushions. I wanted to push or challenge her.

But on the last morning of the program, she suddenly opened up like a flower. The transformation was complete – a new light in the eyes, a different posture and body language, and a remarkable change in her voice and her words. In that moment, I learned something profound about gentleness and non-resistance.

In *The Tao of Leadership*, translated and interpreted by John Heider, there is a chapter on Gentle Interventions [14].

> "Gentle interventions, if they are clear, overcome rigid resistances. If gentleness fails, try yielding or stepping back altogether. When the leader yields, resistance relaxes. Generally speaking, the leader's consciousness sheds more light on what is happening than any number of interventions or explanations. Few leaders realize how much how little will do."

It's a wonderful prescription for healing.

Chapter 4

MIND HOW YOU CARE

As an engineer, turned doctor I have always inclined to concrete thinking and pragmatic approaches to life. I am very practical, resilient, down to earth, and competent. The self-improvement section of the bookstore had nothing to interest me and I was deeply skeptical of the whole genre.

I never read *Don't Sweat the Small Stuff*, *How to Win Friends and Influence People* or *What Color is your Parachute?* For all I know they may be really great books. They sold lots of copies.

But a curious thing happened when I was doing a program in life coaching. My coach asked me to do a very simple exercise each night before going to bed. All I had to do was reflect on the most significant interaction that I had experienced that day, and write a brief description of the event and its significance.

My coach gave me a single sheet of paper divided into eight sections: one for each day of the week and one for an end of week summary. There wasn't room to write much for each day's reflection.

'What's this supposed to prove?' I queried. You can see I gave my coach a hard time.

'Just fill it out each night and bring it back to me next week. I don't want you to have any expectations, just try it and see if you notice anything that happens.'

A lot of the exercises were like that. My logical/analytical brain didn't like open-ended exercises with no apparent purpose. But toward the end of the week, I began to notice a pattern.

At the time I was facing a lot of stress in my job. By the end of the day, the muscles in my neck and shoulders were pretty tense and I'd often have a feeling of pressure in my eyes and a headache that wouldn't shift.

When I spent five minutes reflecting on and writing about the most significant event of the day, the tension in my muscles disappeared. The headache was cured. Just like that. Gone.

I was skeptical at first, then puzzled, and finally amazed. It was a powerful demonstration of how my stress levels were directly related to the contents of my thoughts. It also revealed a profound mind-body connection and a capacity to influence what I believed were involuntary stress reactions.

Many of us are not even aware of the continual self-talk that goes on in our minds. Or if we notice it, we tend to equate ourselves with the voice in our heads. That's me talking.

The very first step of meditation practice is simply to become aware that there is a higher level of being, other than the voice in your head. When you sit still and pay attention, you notice thoughts coming and going in all directions. You can begin to notice the contents of your thoughts and how they influence your emotions, feelings and body reactions.

Learned optimism

Being a thought detective is the essential first step in an extraordinarily helpful strategy called "Learned Optimism" [1].

Dr Martin Seligman, a renowned American psychologist who became the founding father of the positive psychology movement, published a book of this title in 1990. It changed my life.

In 1994 my name was picked in a prize draw and I was given an all-expenses-paid trip to the Annual Scientific Meeting of the Australian and New Zealand College of Anaesthetists in Tasmania. As a senior resident on an anesthesia training scheme, this was the very first time I had attended a professional conference. One of the sessions intrigued me: it was entitled, "The health and wellbeing of anaesthetists".

The speaker introduced "Learned Optimism" and assured the audience the strategies outlined in the book were based on solid research and had been very helpful in his own personal and professional life.

Seligman had an enduring fascination with the mental factors that might promote wellbeing and resilience, rather than the usual approach to mental disorders such as anxiety and depressions. When things happen in our lives, he wrote, we tend to give ourselves a running commentary.

Research showed that different people responded very differently to difficult or challenging events. Some people tended to catastrophize events with self-talk that was negative, pessimistic and self-blaming. Other people, who tended to be more resilient, explained away bad events by blaming external factors.

Seligman called this phenomenon, "Explanatory Style". He showed that the quality of explanatory style – either optimistic or pessimistic – was a powerful predictor of success in almost any life endeavor, whether passing an exam, winning a race, or getting a job.

With research on thousands of subjects, both children and adults, he teased out three different components of explanatory style. He called these the Three P's: Personal, Permanent and Pervasive.

So let's imagine I invited a crowd of mates to a party at my house on Saturday. Only three turn up. The event is a big flop. If I'm a pessimistic thinker, this is the kind of self-talk that goes through my head:

- **Personal:** People didn't come to my party because they don't like me (my explanation blames myself rather than external factors).

- **Permanent:** My social events are always a disaster; probably nobody will come to my birthday next week (bad things keep happening).

- **Pervasive:** I know the team meeting at work on Monday is going to go badly (bad events in one sphere of my life cross-contaminate other aspects of my life)

On the other hand, if I had an optimistic explanatory style, I'd find valid external reasons for the small number of people coming to my party (the Rugby World Cup Final was on at the same time).

I'd quickly forget about my failed party, and I'd feel certain it had nothing to do with my work life.

Seligman advocates becoming a "thought detective", to notice the things we are telling ourselves and to examine if there is any external evidence in support of our self-assertions.

His research showed that many people with a Western upbringing had unrealistically pessimistic explanatory style. When they searched for external evidence in support of their negative thoughts, they couldn't find any.

In a large number of research studies Seligman showed that when you taught people to notice and challenge their thoughts, their performance in a wide range of challenges was significantly improved.

I had always believed I was an optimistic person and when I set my sights on something, I'd rarely fail to achieve my goal. However, when I did the self-assessment questionnaire in "Learned Optimism" I was shocked at the result. My score was well into the pessimistic range, particularly in the Personal domain.

I quickly adopted the practice of learned optimism and have found it immensely helpful in my life. I use it almost every day.

So, for example, I might be trying to do a spinal anesthetic in an older patient. Sometimes the spine is distorted with arthritis and it can be very difficult to get the needle through to the spinal canal.

In previous times, pretty soon I would have been sweating. The thoughts running through my head would be something like, 'You're never going to be able to do this spinal injection (permanent); you already made a mess of the iv line (pervasive); let's face it, you'll never be as good as doctor x (personal).'

Nowadays, I'd be much calmer. I'd be saying to myself, 'Relax, some patient's spines are just really difficult; if you keep calm and try some different approaches, you're bound to succeed; you've done hundreds of difficult spinals before.'

In my experience, many health professional are harshly self-critical, and a few I've met continually sabotage their success in life.

One anesthesiology trainee I knew had finally managed to pass his fellowship exam, after many attempts, and should have been looking forward to a successful career. All he needed to do was organize a one-year fellowship post overseas but he'd received a string of rejections.

His marriage was suffering.

When I talked to him about it, I realized that he was deeply pessimistic about finding a post, he was fearful his marriage was about to break up, and he blamed himself for everything. I knew him to be a competent, careful and thoughtful doctor.

I lent him one of my three battered and stained copies of Learned Optimism – I'd been passing them around among my colleagues. A month later I saw him in the hospital corridor – he looked like a different person!

He was standing taller, had a spark in his eyes, and greeted me enthusiastically. He'd just been appointed to a post in a prestigious teaching hospital. His wife phoned me to express her heartfelt thanks. 'I think that book saved our marriage,' she said.

Being present

The ability to notice and to regulate our thoughts is the first step in managing our minds. Although it often seems that our emotions arise in direct response to life's events, careful self-analysis (and neuro-imaging) shows that every emotion we experience is preceded by a thought.

Our reaction to events is highly dependent on our contextual understanding of the behavior. So if we saw a crazed man screaming and rushing to smash a car windscreen with an iron bar, we'd likely feel frightened and angry. If however we saw that the car driver was trapped inside a burning car, we could understand that the man with the iron bar was running to rescue the driver.

The ability to notice and to regulate our thoughts is the first step in managing our minds

The habitual content of our thoughts has a major impact on our feelings, which extend beyond emotions to include body states, like feeling tense, or shaky. A habitual trap is to get stuck in thoughts about the past, or the future, and not notice what is happening in the present time.

So if we were feeling particularly angry about the way our boss unfairly criticized us at work, we could walk for miles ruminating on angry thoughts without having the slightest awareness of our present surroundings.

While negative thoughts about the past often invoke anger, negative thoughts about the future usually elicit anxiety.

We worry about the challenging patient we have to care for, how our annual review is going to go, how we will pay the mounting bills, and whether little Sarah is going to be unhappy at school today?

In contrast, when we are completely absorbed in a present activity – perhaps looking with awe at a beautiful sunset – we lose all thoughts of the past and the future and slip into a calm, meditative and fully present state. It's what we call "being present".

Working in healthcare offers us deep opportunities to be present in our work, fully absorbed in our caring, and forgetting about our worries or resentments.

When you are fully present, your connection with others is dramatically enhanced. Time stops. Your heart rhythms and brain waves coalesce in a coherent pattern. This is the state in which compassion and loving kindness occur. Not only do you powerfully influence the physiology of your patient, but your own body chemistry changes too.

Muscles relax, heart rate and blood pressure fall, soothing hormones like oxytocin flood your bloodstream, stress hormones dissipate, inflammation is reduced, and restorative body functions are enhanced. At the same time your perceptions and sensitivity are sharpened.

Self criticism and self-compassion

It's my observation that highly self-critical health professionals can also have trouble projecting warmth and compassion towards patients.

While modulating your thoughts is an important and useful first step for building resilience and success, deeper aspects of our mental and emotional functioning come into play in the pathway to positivity, wellbeing, and your capacity for compassionate caring.

Paul Gilbert is a pioneer in compassionate mind therapy, teaching self-compassion to patients with mental health problems. His research shows self-criticism and shame are closely linked to depression [2].

Gilbert says that when things go wrong for people, the self-critical are at increased risk of psychopathology, compared to self-reassurers. His study used self-imagery to explore the mechanisms involved in self-criticism and self-reassurance. His findings show a self-critical trait is associated with ease and clarity in generating hostile and powerful self-critical images, while a self-reassuring trait is associated with ease and clarity of generating warm and supportive images of the self.

Those prone to depression have difficulty with self-reassurance. Thus self-critics may not only suffer from elevated negative feelings, but may also struggle to generate positive self-supportive images and feelings.

One day I was called to intervene when an anesthetic colleague was having difficulty placing an epidural injection in a mother needing pain relief in childbirth. This doctor had lost his cool and was snapping at the patient, demanding that she keep still and saying it was her fault if he couldn't put the epidural in.

Health professionals who are highly self-critical can also have trouble projecting warmth and compassion towards their patients

It was obvious to me that the anesthesiologist was furious with himself for struggling to do the procedure and I could imagine how negative and self-critical were his thoughts, feelings and self-images. In his distress, he was projecting blame onto the patient.

The vulnerable patient, in great pain, exhausted with the labor of childbirth, burst into tears in reaction to this unkind and unprofessional behavior. Her husband, equally sleep deprived, frightened, and on-edge, could barely restrain his anger.

The perception of pain is greatly heightened by fear and anxiety. As health professionals we need to be mindful of the attitude, intentions and spirit we bring to every encounter with patients, particular those who are suffering and in pain.

Learning self-compassion is an important element of our growth as health professionals. When we are kind to ourselves, we tend to project much more warmth and understanding to our patients. And when we judge ourselves less harshly, we are less judgmental about the perceived failings of our patients.

The world authority on self-compassion is Dr Kristin Neff at the University of Texas. On her website (self-compassion.org) you can access introductory guides, video clips, a self-assessment test, meditations and exercises for developing self-compassion, research publications, and everything else you wanted to know on the subject.

Competing systems in our mind

Research shows we have specialized emotional regulation systems that underpin our feelings of reassurance, safeness, and wellbeing [3].

These mechanisms have evolved with attachment systems that register and respond with calming and a sense of wellbeing when we are being cared for. These attachment systems underlie the close bond between mother and baby.

Some people develop with insecure attachment, they experience high shame and self-criticism, and their reassuring emotional regulation system is poorly accessible.

Compassionate mind therapy helps them to experience inner warmth, safeness and soothing.

Within our minds we have competing systems of positive and negative thoughts, competing positive and negative self-representations and emotions, and competing systems of motivation, expressed as either approach or withdrawal.

Positive and negative systems are organized in different parts of the brain and are subject to differential development throughout life.

When we get stuck in pessimistic thinking and critical self-images we are continually reinforcing and growing the neural circuits that support these functions.

If, on the other hand, we direct our attention to positive thoughts, kindness, appreciation, self-compassion and compassion for others, then we grow and strengthen the corresponding brain circuits.

The relative activity in these two competing systems can be detected with brain wave recording or functional MRI scans. The balance can change over time.

Both the negative state and the positive state tend to be self-reinforcing. What that means is that relatively small interventions can tip us out of a negative state into a positive state of flourishing, the basis of Fredrickson's Positivity Ratio [4].

What I find so encouraging is that quite short programs in mind training make a highly significant difference to people's lives, both in patients and in clinicians.

Mind training

Gilbert ran a pilot program of compassionate mind training involving 12 two-hour sessions [5]. The results showed "significant reductions in depression, anxiety, self-criticism, shame, inferiority and submissive behavior. There was also a significant increase in the participants' ability to be self-soothing and focus on feelings of warmth and reassurance for the self."

A pioneering program for primary care physicians in Rochester, New York showed promising results from a similar investment in time [6]. The course included a one day retreat, an eight week intensive phase of 2½ hours per week, and a ten month maintenance phase of 2½ hours per month.

The course was designed to address high levels of distress among the physicians, linked to burnout, attrition and poorer quality of care. It included mindfulness meditation, self-awareness exercises, narratives about meaningful clinical experiences, appreciative interviews, didactic material, and discussion.

The program resulted in both short-term and long-term improvements in mindfulness, emotional exhaustion, depersonalization, empathy, and emotional stability.

A similar trial by Shauna Shapiro and colleagues showed in a randomized, controlled trial that an eight-week program of 2 hour session in mindfulness-based stress reduction (MBSR) reduced stress, and increased quality of life and self-compassion in healthcare professionals [7].

Mindfulness and meditation

So what is mindfulness? Ron Seigel and colleagues at the Institute for Meditation and Psychotherapy offer a great layman's introduction to the subject in their opening chapter in *Clinical Handbook of Mindfulness* [8].

Mindfulness is a central part of 2,500-year-old Buddhist tradition, which encompasses mental qualities of focused awareness, held with deliberate intention, accompanied by non-judgment, acceptance, and compassion.

They quote definitions from various authors including Jon Kabat-Zinn, the foremost pioneer in the therapeutic application of mindfulness [9]. Kabat-Zinn defines mindfulness as "the awareness that emerges through paying attention on purpose, in the present moment, and non-judgmentally to the unfolding of experience moment to moment".

Siegel and colleagues use a stripped-down definition of therapeutic mindfulness: "awareness, of present experience, with acceptance." Mindfulness is not a goal in itself, but is a tool to alleviate suffering and to be more effective in our interventions:

> Through mindfulness, we develop "street smarts" to manage the mind. It helps us to recognize when we also need to cultivate other mental qualities — such as alertness, concentration, loving kindness, and effort — to skillfully alleviate suffering.

> For example, if in meditation we are being self-critical, we may want to add a dose of compassion; if we are feeling lazy, we might want to try to raise the level of energy in the mind or body.

Mindfulness alone is not sufficient to attain happiness, but it provides a solid foundation for the other necessary factors.

In the classical literature, mindfulness was usually discussed in terms of its function, not as a goal in itself. Mindfulness is ultimately part of a project designed to uproot entrenched habits of mind that cause unhappiness, such as the afflictive emotions of anger, envy, or greed, or behaviors that harm ourselves and others.

Mindfulness, to be fully appreciated needs to be experienced, rather than just described. We all have moments of mindfulness but the capacity to hold this state of mind increases with practice.

Most of the time in our busy lives we suffer mindlessness, trapped in endless ruminations about the past, or daydreaming about the future. We can eat food without tasting it, walk without noticing our surroundings, or engage in conversation where all our thoughts are on constructing our reply, not actively paying attention to what is being said.

When we bring compassionate mindfulness to the care of patients, we create a space for healing. We become better attuned to subtle cues, sensing and responding to patients' needs and concerns.

In the cultivation of mindfulness, meditation is an important practice. The simplest forms of meditation ask us to focus attention on an object or sensation, like breathing.

We practice being aware of the focus of our attention, of noticing the distracting thoughts and feelings that pass through our mind, and enhancing our vigilance in the task.

In the beginning we realize that involuntary thoughts assail us from all directions. Siegel and colleagues quote one subject saying, "It was like being locked in a telephone cubicle with a lunatic!"

This is a common difficulty that lessens with practice. When I asked a Tibetan spiritual advisor for advice saying I was troubled because my mind kept jumping about like a monkey when I tried to meditate, he smiled broadly.

He indicated a picture on the wall I hadn't noticed before. It showed a monkey sitting on the back of an elephant.

'See, already, you should be congratulated!' he said, chuckling. 'You have already reached the first stage of enlightenment. Before you began to meditate you didn't know your mind was like a monkey!'

With practice meditation becomes easier, just like any kind of exercise.

When I jumped on my bicycle for the first time in a year, my legs initially felt stiff and sore. Yet within three days of regular rides I was beginning to feel more comfortable, fit and strong again. Exercise with the mind works in the same way.

As you develop the awareness and skills, intruding thoughts become less frequent, it's easier to let go of them, and the periods of stillness increase. It's a good idea to try out different meditation resources – you can buy CD's in the shop or download meditation sound files from the Internet.

We all have different temperaments. I found a set of meditation exercises on a CD where the voice and manner of the teacher help me to be soothed and relaxed. Other family members didn't like his style at all and found teachers they were more comfortable with.

Even a small effort in meditation practice can yield useful results. Although a complete beginner in meditation I've noticed surprising results in terms of body reactions.

Curious to discover if meditation had any effect on my blood pressure, I checked it before starting and was happy enough with the result: 128/70 – not bad for a 55-year old who takes no medication.

After twenty minutes of simple breathing meditation I measured it again: 105/55! That was the blood pressure I had when I was a teenager. What this simple experiment revealed to me is how much we stress our bodies in our reactions to everyday life.

Another body reaction I experienced during meditation reinforced for me the mind-body link. As I explained in the beginning of this chapter, I tend to lock stress and tension into my muscles. I'd been troubled for many months with a pain in my right buttock, which no amount of stretching or exercise would shift. I began to suspect I might have a mild case of sciatica.

One day I did a double session of meditation, going from one twenty minute exercise to another. Halfway through the second exercise I felt the knot of tense muscles in my buttock suddenly release and the pain of three months vanished. This was a lasting result and any time I felt it tensing up again I could do another quick 'treatment'.

Mindfulness is a very personal experience. You can find many books and websites on the subject and I leave you to explore this practice according to your own insights and preferences.

One particular form of meditation relevant to patient care is loving-kindness meditation [10]. It involves using silent mental phrases to focus on the inherent connectedness in the world and our universal desires to be happy and free from suffering.

Its purpose is to cultivate attitudes, intentions, and feelings of love, kindness, and compassion, first for oneself and then for all beings. The typical sequence of loving-kindness meditation includes images of a loved one, then a friend, a neutral person, one's community, a person with whom one has difficulties, then all people, or all beings. The idea is to strengthen compassion both for oneself and others.

When I first read about meditation and mindfulness, I regarded it as an esoteric subject linked with ideas of spiritual perfection, mystical practices, and retreat from the real world. I've come to realize that mindfulness is part of every day life.

When we bring compassionate mindfulness to the care of patients, we create a space for healing

As my connection with patients has deepened, I experience precious moments of stillness, heightened awareness, compassion, and loving-kindness. These practices are meditations in themselves. As we gradually shift our thoughts, feelings and habits to more positive states, we are creating in our brains the same changes that occur with regular meditation.

Meditation doesn't have to imply sitting in a quiet room, separate from the world. We can find meditative states in many activities, going for a walk, contemplating the beauty of birdsong, listening to music, or performing simple tasks mindfully.

One of my contemplative practices is washing dishes. Weird, I know! We have a dishwashing machine but it rarely gets used. Even when we have a dinner party, I like to retreat into the kitchen, sift and organize the dishes and perform a quiet ritual of rinsing, washing and stacking.

Mindfulness in clinical practice

Mindfulness and meditation enhance our capacity for effective patient care in several ways. Research shows that meditation cultivates empathy by reducing stress, increasing self-compassion, and learning to dis-identify with one's own subjective perspective [11]. But we also become more positive role models for our patients in encouraging a more holistic approach to wellbeing.

Mindfulness is a therapeutic intervention with benefits for patients in a wide variety of conditions. Kabat-Zinn and his colleague David Ludwig reviewed the role of mindfulness in medicine in the Journal of the American Medical Association [9].

"Much cardiovascular disease, diabetes, cancer, and other chronic illness is caused or exacerbated by modifiable lifestyle factors, and lifestyle modification constitutes primary or ancillary treatment for most medical conditions.

"An aim of mindfulness practice is to take greater responsibility for one's life choices. Thus, mindfulness may promote a more participatory medicine by engaging and strengthening an individual's internal resources for optimizing health in both prevention of and recovery from illness.

"For intractable disease, meditative techniques that alter and refine awareness may modulate the subjective experience of pain or improve the ability to cope with pain and disability."

Mindfulness training has shown benefits in the treatment of chronic pain, psoriasis, type 2 diabetes, sleep disturbance, attention-deficit hyperactivity disorder, and other conditions. Its application in the treatment of hypertension, myocardial ischemia, inflammatory bowel disease, human immunodeficiency virus, and substance abuse is the subject of major research grants.

Ronald Epstein, in a medical article on "Mindful Practice" wrote;

"Mindful practitioners attend in a nonjudgmental way to their own physical and mental processes during ordinary, everyday tasks. Their critical self-reflection enables physicians to listen attentively to patients' distress, recognize their own errors, refine their technical skills, make evidence-based decisions, and clarify their values so that they can act with compassion, technical competence, presence, and insight" [12].

Epstein listed the characteristics of mindful practice as:

- Active observation of oneself, the patient, and the problem
- Peripheral vision
- Preattentive processing
- Critical curiosity
- Courage to see the world as it is
- Willingness to examine and set aside categories and prejudices
- Adoption of a beginner's mind
- Humility to tolerate awareness of one's areas of incompetence
- Connection between the knower and the known
- Compassion based on insight
- Presence

This humane, sensitive, compassionate and humble account of practice is a world away from the cool, disengaged mode of clinical detachment and objectivity I was taught in medical school. Epstein argues persuasively that mindfulness and compassion both inform and sharpen our technical skills and clinical judgments.

If I was a patient, I know what kind of a doctor I would prefer.

Chapter 5

POSITIVELY HEALTHY

According to the World Health Organization, health is a state of positive physical, mental, and social wellbeing and not merely the absence of disease or infirmity. Yet our healthcare system, obsessed with pharmaceuticals, surgery and procedural medicine, almost entirely ignores the factors that promote positive health and wellbeing.

Does it matter?

In a nine-year longitudinal study of 999 Dutch citizens aged 65 to 85, their degree of optimism or pessimism was highly predictive of mortality from all causes but especially cardiac mortality [1].

The 25% of the study group who were most optimistic had only a quarter of the death rate from cardiac disease, compared with the 25% most pessimistic (0.23 odds ratio).

This remarkable difference in mortality rate persisted when adjusted for age, sex, chronic disease, education, smoking, alcohol consumption, history of cardiovascular disease or hypertension, body mass index, and total cholesterol level.

So even if you smoke, you're overweight, have high cholesterol, high blood pressure and a history of heart disease – your survival is greatly enhanced by positivity and optimism.

In a similar study that examined Seligman's "explanatory style" in 96 survivors of a first heart attack, 15 of the 16 most pessimistic men died of cardiovascular disease over the next decade, while only 5 of the 16 most optimistic died, controlling for major risk factors [2].

In a meta-analysis of thirty follow-up studies on happiness and longevity, Veenhoven found that in healthy populations the effect of happiness is comparable to the difference between smokers and non-smokers [3]. Happiness does not cure illness but it does protect against becoming ill.

The 25% of the study group who were most optimistic had only a quarter of the death rate

While most countries spend a small fortune on smoking prevention, how many have health systems that teach patients how to find positivity and happiness?

Martin Seligman, the founding father of positive psychology makes a powerful argument for the adoption of "Positive Health" as a major public health strategy, quoting multiple studies on the links between positive emotional and psychological health, resilience, and improved physical health outcomes [4].

The pathways of positive health

So how does psychological health affect our physical health? There are multiple mechanisms.

Stress is inherently harmful. The cascading effects of sympatho-adrenal activation causes harmful rises in stress hormones like cortisol, inhibition of immune function, raised blood sugar and lipid levels, raised blood pressure, and even coronary artery spasm.

One study of 115 men with known coronary artery disease videotaped the subjects during an interview and simultaneously monitored the patients for signs of transient myocardial ischaemia, including regional wall motion abnormality [5].

Those subjects who exhibited coronary ischaemia showed significantly more anger expressions and non-enjoyment smiles.

It seems that 'grin and bear it' is a poor strategy in life.

The internal stress in these subjects was sufficient to cause a temporary paralysis of part of the heart muscle and impair pumping function.

In contrast, feelings of loving-kindness actually protect the heart from stress, by reducing blood pressure and also by stimulating mechanisms that reduce inflammation and protect us from oxidative stress.

Inflammatory changes caused by free radicals have long been implicated in organ damage and chronic diseases like atherosclerosis. But oxytocin, a hormone closely linked to affiliative bonding and positive social behavior, can protect us from these harmful effects.

Being kind is good for your health. The flood of oxytocin, released when you have feelings of compassion and loving kindness, attenuates the superoxide activity and inflammatory mediators such as interleukin (IL)-6, in both immune cells and vascular cells [6].

So when you strengthen your heart emotionally you are also helping to protect yourself from the development of coronary atherosclerosis. A loving heart is a healthy heart.

The importance of being kind to yourself

Buddhist teachings help us understand the different components of compassion, called 'The Four Immeasurables' [7]. These qualities are called loving kindness (metta), compassion (karuna), joy (mudita), and equanimity (upekkha). The so-called 'four enemies' of these qualities are hatred, cruelty, jealousy and anxiety.

We can have these feelings in relation to ourselves, or directed to others. So for health and wellbeing, self-compassion is as important as compassion for others; anger directed at self is as damaging as feeling angry with other people.

Kristen Neff says self-compassion involves being open to and moved by one's own suffering, experiencing feelings of caring and kindness toward oneself, taking an understanding, nonjudgmental attitude toward one's inadequacies and failures, and recognizing that one's experience is part of the common human experience [8].

The first component of self-compassion involves treating oneself kindly when things go wrong. So in response to a failure or critical error, self-compassionate people show more kindness, self-reassurance, and self-care, and experience less self-directed anger [9].

Treating oneself kindly can include practical measures such as taking time off work to give oneself a break. Recently I was involved in a tragic case of a sudden maternal death. After attending to the patient's bereaved family and supporting colleagues who were distressed by this event, I took two weeks' leave to give me time to process the grief, loss, and trauma of losing a young patient despite our best efforts.

My wife remarked that this was a much healthier response to tragedy than my previous experience of continuing to work as if nothing had happened, after a patient's death. I was able to articulate my need to recover from the emotional stress of this tragedy and received immediate support from the head of the department, who granted me compassionate leave.

The second component of self-compassion is recognizing our common humanity; that no matter how painful our experiences are, they are part of the common human experience. We are not unique or alone in our suffering, loss, or humiliation.

The third part of self-compassion is mindfulness, taking a balanced perspective of one's situation and not dwelling endlessly in negative emotions.

These kinds of approaches to life are shown to directly affect neuroendocrine, immune and behavioral responses to difficult events. For instance, a six-week trial of compassion meditation, followed by a standardized psychological stress test, showed reduced plasma concentrations of interleukin (IL)-6 and cortisol as well as reduced distress scores [10].

No matter how painful our experiences are, they are part of the common human experience. We are not unique or alone in our suffering

The observed effects were dose-dependent. Those subjects who spent the most time in meditation practice had the greatest reduction in inflammatory markers and also the lowest distress scores in response to psychological provocation.

Compassion-focused imagery stimulates the soothing components of emotional pathways and attenuates hypothalamic-pituitary-adrenal axis activity, with reductions in salivary cortisol [11]. It also stimulates increased heart rate variability, associated with vagal nerve activation and coherence in the heart-brain rhythms.

A short program in mindfulness meditation resulted in enhanced immune response to influenza vaccination. Compared with controls, the subjects who performed an eight-week course in mindfulness meditation had significantly higher antibody levels after vaccination [12].

Similarly, a positive emotional style was shown to dramatically reduce the chances of developing an upper respiratory illness after healthy volunteers were exposed to nose drops containing rhino virus or influenza A virus [13]. The bottom third of subjects with the least positive emotional style were 2.9 times more likely to catch infection than the top third of subjects with the most positive emotional style.

Changing our genetic program

Lifestyle changes including stress reduction and enhanced social relationships may have much more profound effects on our health and longevity. In addition to neural, endocrine and immune changes, such lifestyle changes can radically alter our gene expression, up-regulating protective genes and down-regulating disease-promoting genes.

For too long we have thought of our genetic inheritance as a blueprint that sealed our fate. Now we know that regulation of genes is a highly dynamic process, influenced by many environmental factors throughout our lifetime – a process called epigenetics.

While environmental toxins, exercise, and the quality of our nutrition are important factors, it's the internal environment of beliefs, thoughts and feelings that most powerfully affects our gene expression. The renowned cellular biologist turned crusader, Bruce Lipton, is the leading exponent of epigenetics. I recommend his best-selling book, *The Biology of Belief* [14].

It's almost as if there are multiple possible versions of ourselves, expressed through changes in mental and physical functioning.

Physical fitness, hormonal reactions, inflammatory and stress systems, immune function, nutritional status, and environmental responses modulate our gene expression.

For too long we have thought of our genetic inheritance as a blueprint that sealed our fate

Dean Ornish, the world authority on lifestyle modification of disease processes, has shown that life-threatening disease states can be prevented or even reversed. He advocates a radical lifestyle change involving low-fat diet, moderate exercise, stress reduction, and social support.

Ornish and his colleagues have even reversed coronary artery disease – as demonstrated by coronary angiography – preventing the need for coronary revascularization [15, 16].

Ornish has also shown lifestyle modification can prevent or reverse the progression of low-risk prostate cancer, as assessed by PSA measurement and repeat MRI scans [17, 18].

These research subjects showed multiple changes in prostate cell gene expression with 48 up-regulated and 453 down-regulated genes detected after the three-month lifestyle intervention. These genes are involved in the modulation of biological processes that have critical roles in tumor genesis, including protein metabolism and modification, intracellular protein traffic, and protein phosphorylation.

Perhaps the most extraordinary discovery made by the institute's researchers is that lifestyle changes enhance the activity of telomerase, a crucial protective mechanism in the biology of cellular aging [19].

Telomeres are protective DNA-protein complexes found on the end of chromosomes, which promote chromosomal stability. Telomere shortness is emerging as a marker of disease risk, tumor progression, and premature mortality in many types of cancer, including breast, prostate, colorectal, bladder, head and neck, lung, and renal cell.

Telomere shortening is counteracted by the cellular enzyme telomerase. The lifestyle change program caused an increase in telomerase activity in immune system cells. Furthermore, the degree of telomerase activation was significantly associated with decreases in psychological distress.

So stress doesn't just increase our risk of atherosclerosis but also prematurely ages our cells and increases our risk of cancer. More importantly, investing in lifestyle changes to reduce stress and enhance wellbeing can reverse these dangerous changes.

Health worker stress hurts patients too

Jenny Firth-Cozens is a leading UK authority of stress in doctors. She followed a cohort of 314 medical students through the first ten years of their medical practice, exploring the factors which impacted both physician wellbeing and quality of patient care [20].

Her long-term follow up showed that self-criticism in medical students was a powerful predictor of stress in the years ahead. She recommended programs in cognitive restructuring and psychotherapy for vulnerable individuals.

Since her paper was published in 2001, the advances in positive psychology have given us additional strategies for helping these at-risk individuals.

Rather than treating stress directly, it may be more helpful to enhance wellbeing through measures that enhance work engagement, sense of coherence, self-efficacy, flow and resilience [21]. This is suggested as a fruitful approach in the supervision of psychologists and others who work in inherently difficult and challenging environments such as mental health.

Firth-Cozens showed that stressed physicians are likely to be impaired in their capacity to provide high quality patient care. They made more errors and mistakes, had poor doctor-patient relationships and reduced patient satisfaction.

The reduced trust lessened patients' adherence to instructions and increased the threat of litigation. Stressed physicians had more arguments with colleagues. The physical effects of drug or alcohol abuse also compromised patient care.

One doctor quoted said that he had trouble doing an epidural spinal injection because his hands were shaking so much after a heavy night of drinking.

So health professional stress is not just risky for the individual but it also harms the quality of patient care.

When we feel dissatisfied, stressed and emotionally exhausted we're more likely to perceive that our patients are difficult or make unreasonable demands. We can easily find ourselves in a vicious cycle that often ends in burnout.

The alternative is the positive cycle of flourishing that results when we strengthen our hearts, choose a positive attitude, and find ways to fulfill our aspirations for compassionate, whole-patient care.

The secrets of happy practice

In a report on the Secrets of Physician Satisfaction, by far the highest rating was given to relationship with patients (81%) [22]. The next most important factors were relationships with colleagues (69%), family issues (68%) and personal growth (63%). The lowest rating factor was prestige for role as a physician (49%).

Self-esteem and prestige are shaky foundations for life satisfaction and enduring happiness.

Enhancements in positivity, optimism, mindfulness, sensitivity and compassion don't just benefit our relationships with patients. They are life skills that serve us well in professional and family relationships, leading to significant personal growth.

The research data in the report on physician satisfaction were accompanied by touching quotes from physicians who had found renewed meaning in their practice. One early-career geriatric physician said:

> "I do home visits on my lunch break.... I love seeing patients in their home setting. That is the best way. I started doing home visits, and it healed me. I could relate to what others are going though ... some of the physicians I work with think I am crazy going to the homes. I tell them, you just have to open your eyes. You don't have to be in a box."

The relationship between the health professional and patient is highly interdependent.

Mitchel Adler, writing about the socio-physiology of caring in the doctor-patient relationship found [23]:

1. Empathy is a basic ingredient in a caring relationship
2. A relationship is a mutual, reciprocal engagement, established and maintained by a feedback loop of reactions to reactions
3. Empathy is simultaneously an affective experience and a physiologic state
4. People who influence each others' physiological state can influence each others' health

Adler said the benefits of an empathetic, caring doctor-patient relationship included: Likelihood of a more complete medical history; improved clinical judgment with regard to laboratory tests and procedures; more accurate diagnosis; more cost-effective prescribing; a more satisfied patient who is more informed and adherent to the treatment plan; better treatment outcomes; and reduced physiological stress for the patient, which improves the course of both disease and illness.

Benefits for the physician included greater job satisfaction, less absenteeism, fewer errors, less burnout and less job turnover.

Another study showed that patients' perception of physician empathy strongly predicts patient satisfaction, physician-patient trust and rates of compliance [24].

As a guide to practice, it's useful to consider the qualities measured in the Jefferson Scale of Patient Perceptions of Physician Empathy, used by patients to rate their physicians in the study:

• My doctor understands my emotions, feelings and concerns
• My doctor is an understanding doctor
• My doctor seems concerned about me and my family
• My doctor asks about what is happening in my daily life
• My doctor can view things from my perspective (see things as I see them)

For physicians, personal meaning derived from partnering with patients in their care is inversely correlated with burnout and positively associated with gratitude and professional satisfaction [25].

Empathetic health professionals who make meaningful and personal relationships with their patients have less risk of burnout. The relationship with patients is sustaining, not draining.

The point is reinforced in a recent editorial in the Journal of the American Medical Association (JAMA). Tait Shanafelt MD works at the Department of Medicine Program on Physician Well-being, Mayo Clinic. He said that enhancing meaning in work is a prescription for preventing physician burnout and promoting patient-centered care [26].

Shanafelt quotes the study by Krasner, showing significant improvements in burnout, mood disturbance, empathy, and patient orientation in primary care physicians following a program in mindful communication [27].

Furthermore, he quotes a study where a large medical malpractice insurer developed and tested a stress reduction program for hospital employees that focused on individual training in stress management and organizational control of factors that produced stress.

In a controlled trial that evaluated the longitudinal effect of the program on malpractice claims at 22 participating hospitals relative to 22 matched control hospitals, malpractice claims over the ensuing year were reduced by 70% at intervention hospitals compared with a 3% reduction at control hospitals.

Enhancing meaning in work is a prescription for preventing burnout and promoting patient-centered care

Shanafelt concluded that although many physicians may be tempted to respond to increasing healthcare challenges by taking more time off, by adopting mindful practice they would actually be happier working more.

Krasner's study demonstrated that training physicians in the art of mindful practice had the potential to promote physician health through work.

"Physicians continue to control the most sacred and meaningful aspect of medical practice – the encounter with the patient and the reward that comes from restoring health and relieving suffering."

Meaning in the therapeutic relationship

Creating meaning in the relationship between health professional and patient is therapeutic for patients too. Daniel Moerman and Wayne Jonas wrote a challenging paper entitled, Deconstructing the Placebo Effect and Finding the Meaning Response [28].

They illustrate their argument with the following study:

A group of medical students were asked to participate in a study of two new drugs, one a tranquilizer and the other a stimulant. Each student was given a packet containing either one or two, blue or red tablets. The students were not told that in fact all the tablets were inert and contained no medicine.

After taking the tablets, the students' responses to a questionnaire indicated that the red tablets acted as stimulants while the blue ones acted as depressants; two tablets had more effect than one.

The students were not responding to the inert tablets. Instead, they were responding to the covert "meanings" in the experiment, that red generally means up, hot, or danger, while blue means down, cool, or quiet; and that two will be twice as strong as one.

In another randomized, controlled study, female patients with headaches were allocated to receive one of four medications:

One group had aspirin in a package with a widely advertised brand; the other groups received the same aspirin in a plain package, placebo marked with the same widely advertised brand name, or unmarked placebo.

In this study, branded aspirin worked better than unbranded aspirin, which worked better than branded placebo, which worked better than unbranded placebo.

In commenting on these studies, the authors point out that the "placebo effect" cannot be due to the inert substance in a tablet.

The effect is a result of physiological changes in the patient caused by assigning meaning to the treatment, such as the association of the color red with stimulation, of blue with coolness, and of famous advertised brand with efficacy.

They call this the "meaning response".

Medicine is suffused with meaning, from the white coat of the doctor, her manner and tone of voice, the assumed power of technology, the mystique of medical language, and the doctor's prognosis. Surgery is particularly meaningful and symbolic, with the visible wound, the shedding of blood, and the cutting out of bad things like cancer.

The placebo effect is a result of physiological changes in the patient caused by assigning meaning to the treatment

While the randomized, placebo-controlled trial is the mainstay of measuring efficacy of medicines, the subsequent discounting of the placebo effect as something equating to nothing, not a real effect, is deeply misleading.

The authors plot the distribution of results from 83 randomized, placebo-controlled trials of ranitidine or cimetidine in the treatment of duodenal ulcers. They point out that in the overall distribution of many trials, rates of healing in the treatment group correlate with rates of ulcer healing in the placebo group.

Those studies that had a high healing rate in the treatment group also tended to have a high healing rate in the placebo-controlled group. The authors conclude that the healing response is a combination of the pharmacological action of the drug, and the meaning response of the patient.

In those studies where the scientists infused a deep sense of trust, belief and meaning in the treatment, then both groups, treatment and control, had a high rate of healing.

In many studies, the healing rate in the control (placebo) groups exceeds the healing rate in the treatment group in other studies. Clearly the meaning response is not a nothingness. Placebo sometimes has a greater healing effect than pharmaceutical treatment.

Meaning is conveyed in every interaction with a patient, for good or bad. A friend asking a female breast surgeon about the prognosis for her condition was coldly told 98% of patients with her presentation would be dead within five years.

This pronouncement struck dread in my friend's heart. She fled from the consultation devastated with the lack of emotional support and bitter about the way her hope had been cruelly extinguished. Ten years later she was alive and well – she had found the needed support and healing elsewhere.

A double helix of healing

Compassionate practitioners elicit an equally positive response in their patients. A space of healing is created where both practitioner and patient grow.

Those health professionals who have found their own positive turning point find that their patients respond in different ways. There is a deepening of the meaning in the relationship, a new joy and satisfaction in work and the positive changes are quickly reinforced.

When we humbly serve our patients, they grow in their own capacity to deal with life's misadventures. When we look after our own health and wellbeing, we provide a positive role model for our patients.

Most of the chronic disease we treat in modern healthcare is preventable. If our patients had the encouragement to adopt lifestyle changes, to find ways of flourishing in their own lives, much of the burden on the healthcare system would be reduced.

If we can bring deep empathy, compassion and understanding to our patients then we communicate a healing force that has the power to profoundly affect our patients' physiology, to reduce harmful stress, to boost cellular healing, to heighten immune responses, and even to turn on protective genes.

In the process we also help to heal ourselves.

It's a double upward spiral of healing for both practitioner and patient as we find our own personal path of flourishing.

Chapter 6

CHOOSING TO LOVE YOUR WORK

Since the late 90's I have campaigned for patient safety, investment in clinical leadership, person-centered healthcare, and humane healthcare institutions.

My journey of leadership has been lonely and painful, often at odds with institutional priorities. I have suffered many setbacks and losses. Speaking out about a lack of caring and compassion won me few friends.

So after many setbacks and false starts I eventually discovered there was only one way to change the world. I had to change 'me' first.

It's been a long journey of gradual learning. My greatest teacher proved to be an unforgettable patient I cared for more than fifteen years ago. When I first met Jessie, she was 85 years young. I had the unenviable job of anesthetizing her for major surgery.

Jessie had bowel cancer. She attended the hospital in a wheelchair, looking crumpled and lopsided owing to a devastating stroke she'd suffered twenty years before. Her left side was paralyzed. She was overweight and the tissues of her face sagged in untidy folds like an unmade bed. Jessie had only half a smile but there was mischief and light in her eyes.

Despite an appalling catalogue of medical complaints, she still managed to live alone and I quickly began to sense an indomitable spirit.

Jessie was in big trouble. Her bowel cancer was bleeding and she was very anemic. The tumor was partly obstructing her bowel and it was hard for her to eat. The colicky abdominal pains were troublesome.

In addition to her devastating stroke, Jessie had a long list of serious medical complaints. She had complicated and severe heart disease. Her aortic heart valve was calcified and severely narrowed. Her coronary arteries were clogged. She teetered on the edge of a heart attack and suffered frequent attacks of chest pain.

Her anemia greatly exacerbated her heart condition and she was breathless with a build-up of fluid in her lungs. She also had diabetes, high blood pressure, raised cholesterol and damaged kidneys. Each day, she took eleven different medications in a vain attempt to stabilize her medical condition.

I concluded that Jessie had only a fifty-percent chance of surviving her operation and that her prospects of ever leaving hospital were dismal. There was very little we could do to improve her condition although correction of her anemia with a blood transfusion would reduce the cardiac risk.

With a heavy heart, I did my best to explain to Jessie the enormity of the surgical risk.

'What's the alternative?' she asked.

'If you don't have surgery, the blockage in your bowel will get worse, the bleeding will continue, and you will probably die of heart failure and bowel obstruction.'

'Is there any other form of treatment for the bowel cancer?'

'No,' I replied, shaking my head. 'We would do our best to keep you comfortable.'

'Well, I really don't have a choice then,' she said with determination. 'Robin, I want you to take on my case. I'll take my chance. I've had a good life and if I die having surgery then it's not anyone's fault. I won't blame you.'

I began to explain to Jessie that we could reduce the risk of her surgery if we treated her anemia.

Jessie smiled sweetly and told me she would not be having a transfusion! She saw the expression of dismay on my face.

'Robin, I'm a Jehovah's Witness and can't accept a blood transfusion.'

In a surprising gesture, she took my hand in hers. 'Robin, I put my faith in you. I know you'll do the best job you can and God will be watching over you.'

This was getting very personal and I struggled to maintain what I thought then was the proper clinical detachment. I felt embarrassed and was anxious for this uncomfortable consultation to end.

On the eve of surgery I felt duty bound to explain again the dire risks she was facing. Jessie interrupted my listing of the perils she faced. 'Robin, we've discussed that already. I understand the risks I'm taking but I put my faith in you. I know you will do the best you can.'

She held my hand again saying, 'Robin, you're looking so worried about giving my anesthetic that I think I need to cheer you up. I'm going to tell you a joke!'

Lifting her forefinger up to touch her lips, she blew a lopsided and wet sounding raspberry. 'What's that?' she said!

'I have no idea,' I replied, shaking my head in confusion.

'It's a fart trying to get past a g-string!' she exclaimed with a wicked twinkle in her eye.

I was completely undone. Any semblance of the proper doctor-patient relationship had now dissolved in helpless mirth. When the tears were wiped away, I revised my estimate of her chances of survival. This was a human spirit not yet ready to depart the world. We made our farewell and to my surprise I was able to put aside my fretful worrying to sleep soundly in preparation for the next day's challenge.

Jessie had a stormy time in surgery and post-operative care. She narrowly scraped through several crises, never once complaining. I went to see her again, three days after surgery.

She held my hand again. 'Robin, I prayed that you would survive my anesthetic, and you did!'

Those events took place many years ago. Jessie has since passed on but her spirit stays with me. When I speak at conferences or workshops, I often start my presentation with that story. No other tale has such power to open people's hearts and to remind them why we work in healthcare.

Jessie had many lessons for me but at the time I felt a confusion of thoughts and feelings. For a long time I wasn't open enough to receive her extraordinary wisdom. But hardly a day goes by when I don't reflect on her inspiring example and challenge myself to match her incredible compassion and courage.

Four profound lessons

My wise old teacher had four lessons for me. The first lesson was that of simple humanity.

Jessie, with devastating effectiveness, undid all of my clinical defenses and gave me an experience of shared humanity. She used one of the most powerful tools at our disposal – humor and laughter. It was the start of my journey of personal healing. It's something I try to teach my colleagues, the stepping aside from professional and expert roles to simply be a caring human being.

The second lesson from Jessie was one of interconnection and interdependence.

Before meeting Jessie, I conceived of the doctor-patient relationship as a one-way street. I was the highly trained doctor, the expert, and the person with authority and control. Caring was a one-way process. I cared for patients and I determined the process and the agenda.

Patients didn't care for me. They were grateful, of course, they took my advice and they did what I told them. Those who didn't were 'difficult' patients or 'non-compliant'. We meet such patients in practice every day. They cause us a lot of trouble.

But somehow, Jessie turned the tables on me. She was the one caring for me and supporting me in my vulnerability. The relationship had become a two-way process. At the time, I didn't realize the profound significance of what she had taught me.

I had to undo years of practice to consciously choose a different way of relating to patients.

Jessie's third lesson was that laughter is the best medicine.

No matter how dire the circumstances, there is a place for sharing gentle humor, mischief, fun and a good belly laugh. If we can learn to laugh at ourselves then we open up our hearts to a deeper human connection and the humility to learn. Laughter is a wonderful release for tension and anger. A workplace that creates fun and humor through the daily challenges is a more joyous, creative and energizing place to work.

The last and most important lesson from Jessie was about choosing an attitude.

In the face of severe disability, constant pain and the prospect of almost certain death, Jessie chose to have a positive attitude. She wasn't grumpy or ill tempered. She didn't complain. She didn't dwell on her misfortune. She chose instead to show concern and compassion for me as a vulnerable human being. She gave me support, she cheered me up, and she told me a joke!

If Jessie could choose humor, laughter and compassion in her awful circumstances, then what excuse do we have to be grumpy or feel sorry for ourselves?

Attitude is highly contagious. And attitude exists at many different levels, from the individual, through the team, to the whole organization. We can sense it the moment we walk into a place like a hospital.

The power of choosing your attitude

Some years later I was to learn that choosing an attitude is one of the most powerful ways we can change the world for the better. It was a powerfully liberating experience.

The thought came to me in the small hours of one morning while driving to the hospital to attend a woman in childbirth.

I was exhausted, grumpy, resentful and feeling sorry for myself. After a busy day this was my fourth call of the night.

I had been in bed only ten minutes after the last call-out and was angry that the midwife hadn't contacted me when I was already in the hospital.

This story is about the sometimes-fractured relationship between midwives and hospital specialists. Here are two groups with profoundly different philosophies and experiences.

The midwives come with a strong belief in childbirth, as a natural process for which there should be minimal medical intervention. The hospital specialists see only the clinical crises in childbirth and have to respond swiftly to life-threatening emergencies.

There is an understandable tension between the values and beliefs of these two groups of professionals, resulting in friction, distrust, and mutual blaming.

I carried my resentment into work with me and was occasionally intolerant of frustrations, delays or missing equipment. It wasn't always the friendliest of receptions when I entered the labor room. Sometimes it felt like I was the enemy, the 'wicked' doctor interfering in the natural process of childbirth.

Finding the right equipment, gaining the midwife's help in positioning the patient for the epidural injection, and communicating instructions, felt like an uphill struggle. Sometimes the epidural didn't work well and I'd be called out of bed again.

As I drove into the hospital with all these negative thoughts and feelings, I suddenly felt very ashamed. Jessie's spirit came to me. What right did I have to feel grumpy and sorry for myself when I was being invited to take part in an intimate and life-changing event?

I decided at that moment that every time I was called out I would dispel negative thoughts and instead reflect on the extraordinary privilege of the invitation.

So now I take great care with the spirit and presence I bring to the patient. I enter the labor room softly with compassion and gentleness. I notice how this affects the mother in reducing fear and distress.

I greet and acknowledge the other people in the room. I ask the midwife if she has been busy and when she last had any sleep or rest.

I do the epidural injection with the minimum of fuss and then witness the miracle of pain relief. It is a joyous experience. I don't care how tired I am. I go home with love and joy in my heart.

How amazingly the world changed when I chose to have a different attitude!

Sometimes I thought the midwives resented my coming to do an epidural. Some were surly and uncommunicative, they would neglect to introduce me to the patient or other family members in the room, I would have to ask for assistance, the equipment wouldn't be ready.

Now I feel like an honored visitor. I am greeted warmly. I have the sense that my praises have been sung to the patient even before I step into the labor room. The midwife thoughtfully prepares for my arrival, finding all the equipment and positioning the patient ready for the procedure. I find that the pain relief is more effective and the rate of complications is greatly reduced.

It's as if all the grumpy and difficult midwives have had a personality transplant – and they probably thought the same about me!

For most of my career, I considered the problem of the relationship with midwives as an external problem, a consequence of their difficult attitude and behaviors. My more recent experience leads me to believe that the problem, and certainly the solution, existed in my own head. The only person who changed was 'me' but the consequence of that was a remarkable change in my whole world experience.

Sometimes you have to change 'me' to change the world.

Redefining the professional role

I began to reflect on my professional role, how I might best serve my patients and where I might find the deepest joy and satisfaction. I came to realize that for much of my career, my identity and self-esteem were wrapped up in being a highly trained technical expert.

I was always friendly and helpful but I was certainly the person in charge of the agenda. If my patients had questions, beyond the scope of my technical expertise, I was skilled at diverting them back onto safer ground.

Over time, I have gradually re-conceptualized my role as that of a caring human being first and an expert second. That enabled me to be more humble and respectful, to listen patiently, to form more trusting relationship with my patients and to bring much greater compassion and humanity to the relationship.

I began to take great pleasure in helping patients in whatever way I could, regardless of whether or not it related to my specific technical role as an anesthesiologist.

Over time, I have gradually re-conceptualized my role as that of a caring human being first and an expert second

After all, the complexity of healthcare is bewildering for patients and we have many opportunities to help them navigate the system and find the help they need.

One day, I decided that I would no longer have 'difficult' patients. I decided that difficult patients didn't exist 'out there' but were a consequence of my own judgment or attitudes. The real problem was a difficult doctor, not a difficult patient. I owned the problem, rather than projecting it out. This had an interesting effect.

Most 'difficult' patients have a long and checkered history of interaction with health workers. They have often been judged, blamed, treated with a lack of compassion and even on occasion have been punished by health professionals.

A classic example is the patient with chronic pain admitted to an acute care setting. Often their behavior is interpreted as 'drug seeking'.

When I shifted my attitude to one of compassion and non-judgment, I noticed an immediate effect. Often the patients were surprised or taken aback. They were quite unused to doctors treating them with respect. Many patients ended up crying. Nobody before had really listened to their concerns.

Quite suddenly I found I rarely had difficult patients any more. This was definitely an improvement in the quality of my working day! But paradoxically, the only person who changed was me.

Power to change the world

In our everyday relationships we are constantly trying to interpret and understand others' behavior. Particularly in the Western world, which emphasizes individual freedom and autonomy, we tend to attribute personal behavior to innate characteristics such as personality or motive, rather than situational factors.

However, psychologists have shown that we greatly under-estimate the influence of situational factors on behavior and they call this the Fundamental Attribution Error.

A simple reflection on your own life experience will confirm this bias. For instance, most of my life I have been a shy, introverted and socially unconfident person. But I noticed at work that one nurse in the operating theatre had such a bubbly, cheerful and outgoing personality that in her company I found myself being witty, happy and flirty.

When I observed more closely, I noticed she had this effect on everyone. When I thought about her experience of the workplace, I realized that her everyday reality was a happy, cheerful, sociable place. In contrast, my experience of the same people in the same workplace was much more subdued, quiet and distanced.

When I was teaching interns about the power of choosing a personal attitude, I thought up this parable:

> A man from Mars was sent to Earth to make observations for two weeks. By chance he ended up riding invisibly in the passenger seat of a police car, observing the world 24/7. When he returned to Mars he reported his astonishing finding: Every Earthling drives at exactly the speed limit!! Not just occasionally, but everywhere, all the time!

When I asked my interns to explain this strange observation they eventually figured out that it was the blue and yellow paint on the outside of the police car that had this effect. Every driver within sight of the police car slowed down to the speed limit. Wherever the police car went, it was surrounded by a kind of bubble, in which everyone keeps his or her speed down.

For the man from Mars, this was his total world experience.

So, I said to my interns, 'Be careful what paint you wear on your skin. The attitude you bring to life creates your entire world reality.' The bubbly nurse works in a happy and friendly place where the grumpy surgeon complains that everyone is irritated with him.

In any situation, we have choices about how we respond.

That's what *response-ability* means, the power to respond in an effective way rather than just react emotionally.

So when you are driving to work and some idiot pulls out of a junction right into your path, forcing you to brake suddenly, how do you respond?

Most drivers, struggling through the daily grind of rush hour traffic, react angrily, yell at the driver, toot the horn, and spend the next ten minutes complaining bitterly about stupid drivers.

Or you could choose a different response. Maybe you could reflect on the good fortune that your responses were so swift that you prevented a collision? Maybe you could imagine that the other driver is having a really bad day and was distracted or just made a simple mistake? Better still, you could wave and smile at the other driver.

Our habitual responses can shift over time, if we bring some mindfulness to this task.

> An old Cherokee Indian told his grandson, "My boy, there is a battle between two wolves inside us all. One is Evil. It is anger, jealousy, greed, resentment, inferiority, lies, and ego. The other is Good. It is joy, peace, love, hope, humility, kindness, empathy, and truth."
>
> The boy thought about it, and asked, "Grandfather, which wolf wins?"
>
> The old man quietly replied, "The one you feed."

Vulnerability to negative emotions is thought to lie in memory representations of the self, representing negative self-schemas [1]. These memories are activated by triggering events and maintain negative mood.

But our memory also contains positive self-images. Our thoughts and attitudes affect the competition for retrieval of either positive or negative memory representations and hence influence our mood.

Give it a try. If you are habitually frustrated with your rush-hour commute, decide that today you are going to stop at every junction and let another driver into the queue. Smile and wave. Not only will you arrive at work feeling much more positive but you'll also notice that other drivers become more courteous and let you in to a queue more often.

Surveys of health professionals show that many are unhappy at work, they've lost job satisfaction, they're stressed, and heading for burnout. But here's a question: How much time do you spend rehearsing your unhappiness and activating negative memories?

On my drive into the hospital in the night, after being called out of bed, my mind would habitually be filled with thoughts of self-pity, resentment, grumpiness and fatigue. Many of us spend inordinate amounts of time in self-talk or in conversations with work colleagues about how unhappy we are.

The most powerful way to improve your work experience, to build your wellbeing, happiness and resilience is to CHOOSE TO LOVE YOUR WORK.

Make a deliberate choice about where you focus your attention. Every single day, healthcare offers opportunities for deep pleasure, satisfaction and meaning in the connection with patients and families. Take pleasure in the smallest things. Be mindful of the attitude you bring to each patient encounter.

The latest research from the growing field of positive psychology shows that gratitude and appreciation are two of the most important practices for enhancing positivity, happiness and wellbeing [2]. Appreciation is a habit to be developed, not an inborn personality trait.

Expressing appreciation to others strongly enhances social bonds. When you bring this attitude to your care of patients, you will find that patients respond much more positively, you'll enjoy your work more, and suffer fewer complaints. Teamwork will be enhanced.

Here are some of the things you can appreciate every day:

- The extraordinary privilege of relating to patients and their families in their most intimate and life-changing events
- The resilience and courage of patients in dealing with illness, injury and loss
- The wicked humor of patients like my friend Jessie
- The amazing dedication and kindness of your fellow health professionals
- Little acts of kindness done by others to help your work
- The miracle of healing
- The gratitude of patients and families
- A loving touch
- The mystery and awe of life's purpose
- Relief of pain and suffering

Becoming a champion for compassionate care

There are three powerful strategies in becoming a champion for compassionate care: strengthening your heart; choosing to love your work; and learning the skills so you always find time to care. These three strategies all reinforce each other and allow your compassionate caring to rise above institutional rules and practices.

These strategies are effective in any workplace, no matter how pressured. In every institution there are health professionals who move through the day with grace and ease. They seem immune to the daily vexations and frustrations and find creative ways to serve their patients with love, patience and compassion. This is a state you can achieve too.

The human brain is extremely plastic – in other words, it adapts its structure and function throughout life [3]. When you exercise in the gym, your muscle tone, strength and bulk increase quickly. The same is true of structures in your brain. Positive and negative emotions, and their related motivation systems, are organized on different sides of the brain.

When you exercise the positive emotions of gratitude, appreciation, compassion and loving kindness you cause structural changes to occur in your brain. It's not called "the practice of compassion" for nothing. The centers associated with positive emotions and pro-social behaviors actually grow bigger, create more connections, and increase their blood supply.

Over time you will achieve greater resilience, equanimity, happiness and contentment. Everyday irritations will lose their power to trigger negative emotions. You will become much less prone to disorders of anxiety and depression.

These changes are also associated with significant improvements in physical health including lowered blood pressure, enhanced immune function, and reduced risk of heart disease.

When you choose to love your work, you enhance the health both of your patients and yourself.

Chapter 7

HEALING HANDS

Of all the true stories told by a patient, one I heard at a healthcare quality conference in Australia haunts me the most.

Stuart Diver, a young ski instructor, was the only survivor of the 1997 landslide that tore through the Thredbo ski resort in New South Wales, claiming eighteen lives in the dark and cold. Stuart was trapped under tons of concrete and rubble, helpless to defend himself against the merciless tides of freezing water that drowned his wife Sally, trapped at his side. Stuart was utterly alone for three nights and two days, entombed in wet concrete, rubble and ice, far from help.

On the third day, rescuers lowered listening equipment into the rubble and heard a voice. Paramedic Paul Featherstone crawled down into the rubble and was just able to reach Stuart's hand. For eleven hours he held Stuart's hand and spoke with him, remaining in position even when the rubble shifted dangerously.

When Stuart told his story to the conference, the whole audience shared his tears as he told the story of his wife's death, then being alone for so long. It was hard to imagine that anyone could survive such an ordeal but Stuart let us know that he owed his life to the paramedic who simply gave him hope and comfort for so many hours.

As the last slab of concrete was lifted clear, Stuart's frozen body was lifted out of the wreckage amid the jubilant cries of the rescuers. He was rushed by helicopter to the nearest hospital where the trauma team swiftly began their resuscitation and treatment – so many skilled hands doing so many tasks all at once.

This last experience for Stuart was deeply traumatizing. For the previous eleven hours another human being had held his hand and given him comfort and hope. In the frantic busyness of resuscitation, that human contact was abruptly withdrawn and Stuart lost all hope.

Choking back the tears, Stuart told the stunned audience that the experience of resuscitation in the hospital was worse than his wife dying and worse than being entombed. Few could ever calibrate human suffering with such poignancy.

For our patients, illness and injury often hit like a landslide. They find themselves trapped and alone. Our caring touch might be the only thing that gives hope and comfort. When we touch our patients, they touch us in turn. These precious moments let us know we are not alone in our fear and suffering, either as patients or professionals.

Non-clinical touch

In medical school I was taught touch as a scientific instrument: palpating the abdomen, percussing the chest, feeling the pulse, sensing the apex beat of the heart, testing for muscular strength, feeling the texture of a rash on the skin, testing for edema. The emphasis was clinical, impersonal touching.

Touch as a therapeutic modality, a means for human connection, or to offer comfort and caring was completely off the syllabus. Sometimes it seemed that avoidance of touch was necessary to maintain the proper clinical detachment. Other times it felt like touch might be dangerous, that the affliction of a dying patient might be somehow contagious.

Patients at the end of life talking about the elements of care spoke of the importance of touch [1]. They felt that their illness separated them from staff and recommended touch as a way to communicate and overcome this separation.

"Maybe a touch on the shoulder… not a feeling of intimacy but of friendship… it makes a big difference."

"Touch the patient; you will not get the disease, you should know better. You will not die if I am dying and you squeeze my hand or say something nice."

Touch is an essential component of providing comfort but the usual nursing and medical protocols for patient care only recognize a neutral sense of comfort as in the absence of a specific discomfort, not as a positive construct.

Kolcaba suggests that we need to appreciate comfort as a positive, holistic outcome and created a framework for 'Comfort Theory' in pediatric nursing [2].

For our patients, illness and injury often hit like a landslide. Our caring touch might be the only thing that gives hope and comfort

A loving touch can offer exquisite comfort to a frightened, suffering or bereaved patient. While some people are comforted and reassured with words, others are much more powerfully affected by touch.

I grew up in a culture where physical displays of affection were taboo. When my parents left me at boarding school at the age of ten, their farewell was a handshake, not a hug and a kiss. As an adult I had to learn from the beginning how to convey feelings through touch. But I am also profoundly 'touched' when people offer me physical comfort, even just a light touch on the arm.

In the healthcare setting we can convey concern through touch, in ways universally recognized across many cultures. We can add extra warmth to a handshake by adding our second hand. Many patients are deeply grateful for the comfort of a hand held quietly, for instance during a procedure that causes them anxiety. Or else we can simply lay our hand on top of the patient's hand without having to hold it.

Empathy and concern are conveyed by a light touch to the upper arm or shoulder, a universally recognized and unambiguous gesture.

It's a good idea to avoid patting the patient. I recall seeing a gynecologist patting my wife on the knee during a clinic appointment. It was intended as a gesture of reassurance but it felt patronizing, as if she were a dog or small child to be petted.

The healing power of a hug

I've met patients who say a hug from their doctor left them profoundly moved and created a cherished memory for a lifetime. When patients or family members are lost, afraid, grieving, or suffering, a simple physical gesture of comfort can have a powerful impact.

At a recent conference in Australia, I ran a small workshop for twelve participants using appreciative inquiry to explore "peak experiences" of compassionate caring. Participants interviewed each other in pairs and then shared their stories with the whole group. The experience was so moving that these twelve strangers all hugged each other and shared tears.

A male general practitioner, relating an event that occurred twenty or even thirty years before, told one of the stories. In the Australian culture of the time, there had been a strong taboo against any display of emotion or vulnerability by the male of the species!

His patient, a retired bank manager in his seventies, visited often, complaining of chronic back pain. Reading between the lines, the wise doctor sensed the real problem was loneliness and a loveless marriage.

One day, the patient stood up to exit the consulting room but paused before the door saying, 'I think I need a hug.' His startled doctor responded to this invitation.

When the old general practitioner told this story to the group, tears ran down his cheeks. This hug was the first time he had ever offered physical comfort to a patient. It profoundly affected his practice and opened up a whole new way of relating to patients.

So learning to touch and to offer physical comfort to our patients is healing to both parties. Our empathy allows us to feel the suffering of our patients and can cause us distress. But when we bring openhearted compassion to the relationship, the barriers between practitioner and patient dissolve and we can comfort each other. The hug is as much for the nurse or doctor as it is for the patient.

Making the human connection

Researchers have explored these issues by observing and analyzing the detail of the patient-practitioner interaction. A synthesis of the research on modes of touching in nursing care concluded that nurses employ two quite different ways of relating to patients: a contact and a connection [3].

In a contact the nurse is using task-oriented touch and is present as being there for the patient. The nurse and the patient are relying on roles that limit the degree of interpersonal connection.

In a connection the nurse is listening, using caring and connective touch and is present as being with the patient. Connection is grounded in mutual receiving, which allows a high degree of interpersonal connection. The nurse and the patient are not only present to each other as roles but also as unique persons.

The healing power of touch

There is overwhelming scientific evidence touch can affect patients' healing and recovery by modulating stress response, immune function, pain perception, and physiological parameters.

Therapeutic Touch (TT) is a complementary therapy where the practitioner places hands close to the patient – usually without touching – and focuses a strong healing intention.

In randomized controlled trails, Therapeutic Touch has:

- Reduced pain and cortisol levels, and enhanced Natural Killer Cell function in post-operative patients [4]

- Enhanced parasympathetic nerve function, reduce complications and length of hospital stay in premature infants [5,6]

- Reduced pain in multiple independant clinical studies (meta-analysis) [7]

- Reduced fatigue and pain levels in chemotherapy patients [8]

- Reduced anxiety levels in pregnant inpatients withdrawing from drug dependency [9]

- Reduced restlessness and variability in cortisol levels in nursing home residents with dementia [10]

- Increased hemoglobin levels and hematocrit in students with anaemia [11]

- Reduced pain scores, lessened depressive symptoms, and improved sleep quality in patients with chronic pain [12]

Other types of therapeutic massage and healing touch have also shown benefits. In a randomized, prospective, crossover trial of patients receiving cancer chemotherapy, they lowered blood pressure, respiratory rate and heart rate [13]. These therapies also lowered anxiety, fatigue and mood disturbance. Pain ratings were decreased and four-week analgesic drug use was reduced.

The effects of therapeutic touch can even be demonstrated in tissue cultures, suggesting a direct impact on cellular function. In a controlled trial of human tissue cells in culture – fibroblasts, tendon cells (tenocytes), and bone cells (osteoblasts) – cultures which were exposed to therapeutic touch showed greater proliferation and DNA synthesis [14].

Even more intriguing, therapeutic touch may have a direct cellular effect in suppressing the growth of cancer cells and enhancing the differentiation of normal cells.

In tissue culture studies, therapeutic touch appears to increase human osteoblast DNA synthesis, differentiation and mineralization, and decrease differentiation and mineralization in a human osteosarcoma-derived cell line [15, 16].

We don't currently know the mechanism for the physical benefits of touch but the studies on cell cultures suggests there is an energy field extending from the hands of the practitioner that can influence cellular function.

One potential candidate for such an energy field is the electromagnetic field of the heartbeat. Whenever we record the patients EKG (electrocardiogram), we are picking up the electrical energy of the heartbeat on the surface of the body. However, the electromagnetic field of the human heartbeat extends some distance beyond the body and can be detected with sensitive magnetometers.

This heartbeat energy field is powerful enough to affect the firing of brain cells in another person we are touching or in close proximity to. If the EKG is recorded in one subject and the EEG (brainwaves, electroencephalogram) in the second subject, you can demonstrate that some of the brainwaves are precisely synchronized with the first person's heartbeat [17].

When I learned physiology at medical school, the heart was believed to be the passive recipient of controlling signals from the brainstem, to make it go faster or slower, to beat harder or softer. Now we know that the heart has its own nervous system comprising about 40,000 neurons.

The heart is a sense organ continually sending signals back to the brain, directly via the vagus nerve, through the excretion of peptide hormones, and directly by the powerful electromagnetic field of the heartbeat.

Through feelings of loving kindness and compassion, the heart exerts a modulating effect on brain function leading to mental calmness, reduction in stress, and physiological coherence

The heart is often understood as the seat of the emotions. We talk about 'heartache', a 'heartfelt' connection and a 'broken heart'. Research shows that when we have feelings of loving kindness and compassion, the heart exerts a modulating effect on brain function leading to a state of mental calmness, reduction in stress, and physiological coherence.

This latest scientific research accords with ancient Buddhist wisdom. In Buddhist tradition all the negative emotions, such as anger and anxiety, are seen as 'afflictive' emotions that distort our perception and give us an unrealistic view of the world. For instance, when we are in the grip of anger, we tend to demonize the other person, to exaggerate their faults and to ignore their good features.

In Buddhist philosophy, the only mental state that allows us a clear and undistorted perception of the world is openhearted compassion.

When we bring the qualities of openhearted compassion to the care of our patients, we also radiate a healing energy.

Through the power of our touch we can offer profound comfort, reduce pain and stress, reduce anxiety, and stimulate healing at a cellular level.

These actions are also deeply healing for our own bodies.

Gloves Off

One final note on touching our patients: The very real concern about cross-infection of hospital patients, and the emergence of multi-resistant bugs like MRSA, has prompted many of us to isolate ourselves from patients with gloves, gowns and masks.

Working as an anesthesiologist I routinely wear gloves in the operating room, whenever I touch a patient. But holding a patient's hand with a gloved hand is just not the same as bare skin-to-skin contact.

While being mindful of the risk of transmitting infection, we can also choose times when bare skin contact is safe and beneficial.

The widespread availability of alcohol hand rub has made disinfection of hands very quick and easy, before and after patient contact.

The contrast between warm human contact and the sterile clinical performance of tasks is illustrated in a story told by Dr Rachel Remen in her book, Kitchen Table Wisdom – Stories That Heal [18].

At age twenty-nine, Remen had a total colectomy and ileostomy for Crohn's Disease, an illness she had endured since her teens.

After surgery, Remen was unable to change the ileostomy bag herself. Nurse specialists entered her room, donned apron, mask and gloves, performed the procedure, stripped off all the protective clothing, and then carefully washed their hands.

Remen explains that this daily ritual made her feel shamed and untouchable.

One day a beautifully dressed nurse in a silk dress and heels came into her room and asked if Remen was ready to have her ileostomy changed.

Carefully washing her hands before the procedure, she quickly and naturally changed the bag using her bare hands. Remen describes how soft and beautiful her hands were, the pale pink nail polish and gold rings.

Remen's account of this event is vividly described and conveys the huge emotional impact of a nurse willing to touch her in such a natural way. It was the beginning of hope and healing.

When we fully accept the human condition we can bring deeper compassion to the care of patients.

When I go to the toilet at home, I don't wear rubber gloves. I accept there are aspects of body function that are messy, smelly and unpleasant.

Too often we wear gloves and gowns, not because of risk of infection, but because we feel disgusted with the body functions of our patients.

When we accept those things as part of ourselves, then we can touch our patients with grace and ease, like the angel who visited Remen that day and gave her so much healing.

Chapter 8

THE NEUROSCIENCE OF COMPASSION

A close friend of mine, only forty-six years old, developed strange muscle cramps and then realized one day that his hands were getting weak. He could no longer twist the lid off a jam jar. After a bunch of nerve tests and scans he went to see the neurology specialist.

The news was devastating. He had motor neuron disease, an incurable and progressive form of paralysis with an average life expectancy of three to five years. There is no known treatment.

'So how can you help me?' pleaded my friend.

'I'm sorry, there's nothing I can do.'

'So when will I see you again?'

'There's no point in making another appointment. There's nothing I can offer. When you are dying and need palliative care, we can help arrange that.'

'But don't you care?' exclaimed my friend in desperation.

'Look, I have seventy patients on my list with incurable neurological disease. If I spent all my time seeing them I'd never get any real work done.'

My friend stumbled from the consulting room feeling absolutely devastated, alone, and devoid of hope.

'Where was the compassion?' he asked me, with a haunted look in his eyes.

If the doctor and the patient had been wired up with instruments to examine brain function during this painful exchange, we'd have learned a lot about the richness of human communication. No matter how hard the neurologist tried to remain detached, an intimate exchange took place.

The latest advances in neuroscience paint a rich picture of the deep interconnection between human beings: our feelings, sensations, thoughts, emotions, physiological responses, and visceral reactions are intimately linked. It's as if we have a broadband network connection between our respective nervous systems.

Our neurodevelopment, from earliest life to old age, is continually shaped by our interactions with others. So powerful and dynamic is this relationship that a whole new field of science has begun to emerge: interpersonal neurobiology.

Mirror neurons and the science of empathy

The first inkling of such a profound interconnect began with the discovery of mirror neurons, specialized cells in our brain programmed to recognize facial expression, emotional displays, and intention of others. Like many scientific breakthroughs, the discovery occurred by accident.

Neuroscientists were trying to understand the neural basis of voluntary movement. When a monkey sees a piece of banana on the table, how do the neural circuits link an executive intention – picking up a piece of tasty food – with the complex synchronization of many muscles to perform the action?

The researchers found neurons in the pre-motor cortex of monkeys respond to the execution of hand-object interactions [1]. Every time the monkey reached for a new piece of banana, a single large neuron was seen firing on the screen of its recording apparatus.

The latest advances in neuroscience paint a rich picture of the deep interconnection between human beings

One day, the researchers happened to have two monkeys at the same bench, both wired to record signals from the mirror neuron. When the first reached out to take a piece of banana, the monitor connected to the second monkey gave a blip. The startled researchers soon discovered the mirror neurons fired, not only when a monkey performed the action but also when observing another monkey doing the same task.

Within a short time, scientists realized that the motor neuron system allowed individuals to understand others' actions and intentions.

Similar systems of mirror neurons were found that encoded facial expressions and emotional responses – the basis for empathy. When one monkey showed a facial expression of pain, the second monkey showed immediate activation of brain centers associated with painful stimulus. Moreover, there was mirroring in facial expressions and display of emotions between the two monkeys.

Although we can't easily put electrodes in the brains of human subjects, there is substantial evidence from functional MRI scans and other research tools that humans also have a powerful mirror neuron system, allowing us to empathize with others [2].

So sensitive are these circuits that even subliminal images of facial expressions can trigger a response in the observer. When a photograph of a face displaying emotion is flashed on a computer screen for only 1/20 of a second, corresponding movements in the facial muscle of the observer can be recorded. Such extreme sensitivity to the facial expressions of others, even at an unconscious level, is the basis of the intuitive feelings we have about others.

When we develop as adults, we learn to modulate our reactions to different situations and to conceal our feelings. So when someone acts aggressively towards us, we can remain calm and keep our expression neutral. However, we have a fleeting involuntary response to the provocation, displayed as a "micro-expression" – a tiny twitch of the facial muscles that may betray our real feelings.

The responses of the mirror neuron system also include a wide range of somatic and visceral reactions. When we see someone displaying an expression of disgust and retching, we feel nauseated and may even begin to retch ourselves. When we watch athletes performing the high jump on a TV broadcast of the Olympics, our legs involuntarily twitch. When we are close to someone aroused and excited, our own heart rate, breathing and blood pressure increase in tandem.

In one famous experiment involving romantic couples, the female partner was placed in a MRI scanner and the male was threatened with a painful stimulus [2]. The female partner was told that every time a particular symbol appeared on the computer screen, her partner was being hurt. When the symbol appeared, the MRI scan showed activation of her pain circuits, identical to the response she showed when given a painful stimulus directly. We truly feel others' pain.

Sharing physiology

People engaged in meaningful interaction literally share their physiology. This new field of sociophysiology was first demonstrated in 1955 by making simultaneous recordings of affective interactions and physiologic activity of both therapist and patients during psychotherapeutic interviews [3].

This effect is enhanced by the vulnerability of the patient and the emotional availability of the therapist.

Psychotherapy works because it induces long-term changes in the structure and function of the patient's brain, analogous to the neurodevelopment of an infant's brain in the close bond of maternal love. For a fascinating exploration of interpersonal neurobiology, I recommend the book *MindSight: the new science of personal transformation* by Daniel Siegel [4].

Empathy is simultaneously an affective experience and a physiologic state. When we influence the physiology of our patients, we affect their health, for better or worse.

Our physical responses to the experience of others includes reactions in the autonomic nervous and endocrine systems, and hypothalamic-pituitary-adrenal axis regulating body state, emotion and reactivity [5].

This cascade of reactions influences our immune system. In another experiment, researchers showed that a five minute experience of either compassion or anger significantly changed the level of IgA antibodies in saliva [6].

Our emotional displays are highly contagious; they infect others around us. They are powerfully conveyed by our facial expression, the quality of our smile, the tone of voice, and our body language. When we are mindfully present, calm and compassionate, we radiate a powerful field that reassures, comforts and calms others.

We observe this from time to time in everyday life. Some people have an extraordinary presence that can compel attention and calm down a room full of agitated people, even before they utter a single word. Often this ability mirrors an inner stillness.

In medical school we were taught clinical detachment and objectivity as high ideals. Our teachers were role models for an impersonal approach to care where patients were objectified as 'the appendix on ward six' or 'the breast cancer on ward nine'.

When we stood around the bedside on a teaching round, all the talk was about symptoms, signs, investigations, differential diagnosis, and treatment. It was as if the person in the patient hardly existed.

But clinical detachment is a folly. The neuroscience tells us that human beings are profoundly interconnected.

Even if the practitioner believes they are insulated from the emotional threat posed by the patient's suffering, the vulnerable patient is wide open to the emotional impact of the practitioner's behavior.

When we are mindfully present, calm and compassionate, we radiate a powerful field that reassures, comforts and calms others

I have met many patients who felt shocked and angry, and were devastated by the apparent coldness and indifference of health professionals, like my friend with the new diagnosis of motor neuron disease.

Patients don't have clinical detachment to fall back on.

The implications for our clinical work are important. The spirit we bring to our work contaminates all of our patients and our teammates.

When we are grumpy, intolerant, resentful, fatigued and unhappy, we infect others with those feelings. When we are lighthearted, open, happy, caring and compassionate, we help heal those around us.

Many of us are very practiced in the art of conveying busyness. The quick movements, brisk attention to clinical tasks, lack of eye contact, and clipped speech all portray a powerful message: I'm here for you in a strictly limited role, I'm not going to connect with you, and I don't have time for questions or concerns.

The manner in which we reveal our mental state and attitudes are almost completely non-verbal – our facial expressions, tone of voice, eye contact, and body language. This means that we have all the time in the world to convey an attitude of care, kindness and compassion even when we are busy performing clinical tasks.

The kindly nurse doesn't take any longer to check the pulse and blood pressure, administer the medications, adjust the drip, re-do the dressings, and write the chart than the brisk, unfeeling nurse. But by her smiles, eye contact, gentleness, touch and caress she conveys loving kindness.

Recent developments in neuroscience have given us new insights into the complex nature of empathy. The process of empathy includes the bottom-up processing of emotional signals, cognitive appraisal and understanding, and top-down modulations depending on the perceiver's motivation, intentions and attitude [5].

Developmental studies of children imply that distinct but interacting brain circuits serve these different components, which develop at different ages.

Empathy is feeling-with another person where emotions are mirrored whereas sympathy is more a feeling-for the other person.

When you feel sympathy for a sad person, you don't necessarily feel sad yourself; you might instead feel pity or compassion.

Empathy, the ability to intuit and recognize feelings in others, is not necessarily a force for good.

Conmen use skills in empathy to build the trust of their victims. And understanding the suffering of our enemies may cause us satisfaction rather than sympathy.

While empathy is an essential component of compassion, empathy alone is not enough. Empathy does not always lead to compassion, even in the well motivated.

Compassion is defined as the humane quality of understanding suffering in others, combined with a motivation to relieve that suffering. When we witness a patient suffering, our empathy can lead to personal distress, which if too intense can overwhelm our desire to help. We then tend to withdraw rather than show a compassionate response.

This situation particularly arises when health professionals feel there is nothing more they can do to help a patient. If your professional role is limited to technical treatments and you have run out of remedies, the patients' suffering is hard to bear because you feel incompetent and helpless.

Compassion is defined as the humane quality of understanding suffering in others, combined with a motivation to relieve that suffering

Even worse is the situation where your mistake has caused the patient some harm.

Earlier in my career, I can think of a number of patients whom I simply abandoned after making an error – it was too painful for me to witness their distress and face up to my guilt.

Social psychology studies suggest that the ability to focus on the feelings and thought of others promotes empathic concern and altruistic motivation, while a disposition to imagine oneself in the other's distressful situation results in heightened personal distress and an egoistic motivation to reduce that distress by withdrawal.

So while empathy, sensitivity, and a motivation to help are all essential parts of compassion, so too is the ability to tolerate distress within our self.

Competing systems of motivation

The advances in neuroscience demonstrate that how we respond to a given situation depends of the balance between two competing systems of motivation in our brains: an approach system and a withdrawal system [7].

The approach system is organized in the left pre-frontal area of the brain and is associated with positive emotions of love, security and happiness.

The withdrawal system is organized on the right side and is associated with negative emotions such as anxiety, depression, and sadness [8].

Thus the socially insecure person at a party (like me at a younger age), being fearful of rejection or embarrassment, hangs back in the corner and tends not to engage with others – the withdrawal motive wins. The confident partygoer plunges straight into the crowd – the approach motivation in action.

When we respond to a challenging situation, our response depends on the balance of activity in these two competing systems.

If we feel overwhelmed and threatened, we tend to withdraw. If we have greater stores of love and positivity, we find the inner resources to approach the situation and engage.

When we witness a patient's suffering, our empathy causes us to suffer with the patient. So to practice compassion, we must be able to tolerate our distress, stay with it, avoid withdrawing and to offer ourselves in love and support – the approach motivation wins over withdrawal [7].

If we don't have adequate internal resources, we cannot tolerate the distress and we choose detachment. Compassion is lost.

The practices that strengthen the heart, that allow us to maintain compassion in the face of distress, are the daily practices of kindness, gratitude, appreciation and mindfulness.

The scientific evidence shows that regular practice causes structural changes in the brain that enhance and strengthen our positive emotions.

The practices that strengthen the heart, that allow us to maintain compassion in the face of distress, are the daily practices of kindness, gratitude, appreciation and mindfulness

The emotions we habitually engage reinforce the corresponding brain centers – just the same way muscles respond to regular exercise.

When stuck in depression, anger and misery we continually reinforce the neuronal connections in the corresponding parts of our brain, growing new neurons and increasing the blood supply.

On the other hand, if we acquire new habits of kindness, compassion, gratitude and appreciation, we strengthen and grow the parts of the brain that support these positive affects. This is the neural basis for the 'Positivity ratio' discovered by Fredrickson and others working in the field of positive psychology [9].

The relative amount of activity in brain centers associated with positive and negative affect is predictive of our temperament. Those who have grown and developed their positive centers have greater equanimity. The irritations of everyday life don't affect their good mood. These are the people who move through life with serenity.

Neural correlates of compassion

Compassion is associated with a particular pattern of autonomic nerve system response characterized by a dampening down of the 'fight or flight' sympatho-adrenal response and an enhancement of parasympathetic vagal nerve activity accompanied by slowing of the heartbeat.

('Sympathetic' and 'parasympathetic' are technical terms for different arms of the autonomic nervous system that regulate organ function, and don't imply the emotion of sympathy.)

The parasympathetic vagus nerve and associated circuits connect to the 'social engagement system', which includes facial and vocal displays, looking and listening activities, and motor behaviours such as tactile contact – all pro-social behaviours.

The relative activities of the sympathetic and parasympathetic nervous systems can be inferred from rhythmic variations of the heart rate. When the heart rate is plotted against time, sympathetic activation shows up as a disordered and spiky variation in the heart rate with high frequency components. On the other hand, heartfelt feelings of gratitude and compassion are associated with a smooth and rhythmic variation of heart rate and vagal nerve activation.

This smoothed and enhanced pattern of rhythmic heart rate variation correlates with greater sympathy and compassion, less self-reported distress, fewer facial displays of distress and gaze aversion, and less arousal as measured by skin conductance [7].

Similar physiological patterns are seen when subjects practice mindfulness meditation or compassion meditation. Even a short program in mindfulness meditation creates a measurable increase in left-sided anterior brain activation, compared to non-meditators, a pattern associated with positive feelings [10].

In the same research subjects, meditators developed higher antibody levels after influenza vaccination than non-meditators and the magnitude of increase in left-sided brain activation correlated with the boost to immune function.

Functional MRI studies of novice and expert meditators show that the mental expertise to cultivate positive emotions alters the activation of circuitries previously linked to empathy [11]. During a compassion meditation, expert mediators showed a greater activation than novices, suggesting long-term structural changes.

The same researchers have shown both short-term and long-term changes in the brain function of Buddhist meditators, associated with high-amplitude gamma synchrony on EEG recordings [12].

Self-compassion and empathy are closely linked to mindfulness. Programs in mindfulness-based stress reduction (MBSR) show reductions in symptoms of stress and mood disturbance accompanied by increases in mindfulness, spirituality and empathy [13]. While there was no change in the degree of empathic concern, the subjects' response was healthier in terms of increases in perspective taking ('other' focus) and a reduction in personal distress.

While self-criticism activates brain circuits involved in error processing and inhibition, self-reassurance activates quite different parts of the brain linked to compassion and empathy [14]. Self-compassion is shown to be a crucial strategy in promoting positivity, wellbeing and the capacity for compassionate caring.

Does the development of our 'happy' brain circuits mean we are less sensitive to suffering? No - quite the opposite. People who have developed their positivity, empathy and compassion can be exquisitely sensitive to the suffering of others but they show much more rapid recovery from emotional challenge.

One study showed that mindfulness training alters the neural expression of sadness, heightening the visceral and somatosensory representation of emotion – the subjects had a more powerful physical representation of emotion and this seemed to protect against depression. They 'felt' the sadness and then let go of it [15].

Detachment or non-attachment?

Buddhist philosophy offers an alternative to the idea of clinical detachment. In the Buddhist world, cognition and emotion are inseparable. Only in the Western world do we have this strange dualistic idea that intellect and emotion can be separated.

When Western scientists and Tibetan Buddhists first met in a cross cultural exploration of the meaning and function of emotions, sudden difficulty arose in translation [16]. In the Tibetan language, there is no equivalent of the English word 'emotion'. The neuroscientists at the meeting were fascinated with this observation – in their brain scans of multiple subjects they had failed to find a biological equivalent of rational objectivity. In every subject, the cognitive and emotional centers lit up simultaneously.

Studies of brain-damaged subjects confirm this finding. Patients with lesions in their emotional circuitry have profound difficulty making decisions, even though their logical faculties are intact [17].

So if clinical detachment and objectivity are questionable qualities, how do we manage the many competing demands on our attention and still care best for patients?

At times we do need a singular focus on the tasks of care. For instance when I am involved in the urgent resuscitation of a severely injured patient, I cannot afford to be distracted by the emotional implications of suffering, injury and loss.

In Chapter 4, *Mind How You Care*, I explored aspects of mindfulness and the ability to purposely direct attention.

When we are skilled in these practices we can bring a razor-sharp focus to important tasks at one moment, and give our full-hearted compassion the next. Anxiety and fear are the things that most get in the way of this mindful attention to what is needed in the moment.

In Buddhist practice, all the negative emotions are seen as 'afflictive' or 'obscuring' mental states: in the grip of these emotions we are unable to perceive the world without distortion. In contrast, the only mental state associated with clear perception is openhearted compassion.

Buddhist teachings emphasize openhearted compassion combined with a strategy of non-attachment. Unlike the cold, indifferent feeling of Western detachment, openhearted compassion with non-attachment allows one to care with deep compassion and concern.

The non-attachment means that we don't invest in the outcome of our efforts or try to change the things beyond our sphere of influence; we simply do our very best and accept the outcome.

His Holiness the Dalai Lama powerfully embodies this practice. If he meets a beggar on the street, he will stop, offer his prayer and blessings, and maybe shed a tear for the suffering of the beggar. He then walks away knowing that it is impractical to save every beggar by his personal efforts.

However, from the clarity of his openhearted compassion and deep understanding, he devotes his life to practical strategies for reducing suffering in the world.

From a Western perspective of professional responsibility and heroically striving to save our patients, non-attachment is a hard concept to grasp. Eventually we come to understand that our efforts pale into insignificance compared with the capacity for healing contained within our patients.

When we humbly serve our patients, we know that we can only do our best. Most outcomes are far beyond our control.

All of us working in healthcare experience awful tragedy and loss. I have learned to open my heart, connect to the suffering patient, share tears and hugs, and do the best I can to promote recovery and healing. Then I walk away.

Every act of compassion is also an act of self-healing. The pain of witnessing suffering and loss is ameliorated by the deep satisfaction of knowing that your caring made a huge difference to the patient. In the end we are all imperfect and vulnerable.

The therapeutic connection

Beyond all of the wonderful treatments modern medicine has to offer, the most profound healing comes from a bond of shared humanity.

The contribution of neuroscience is to remind us that we are intimately connected with others. To pretend otherwise is to deny our humanity.

We can use this deep connection to profoundly alter our patient's physiology and elicit healing responses. The power of suggestion is something you can easily use in everyday practice, with great therapeutic benefit.

An anesthetic colleague in Adelaide, who is also a trained hypnotherapist, is a master at using suggestion to help patients overcome fears.

One of his patients was a six-year-old boy who came into hospital each month to receive a drug infusion. He had a congenital deficiency in his immune system and needed regular treatment with immunoglobulin.

This poor boy had become terrified of needles. The monthly hospital visit had become so traumatic that the only way to get the needle in the vein was first to administer a general anesthetic by forcibly holding a gas mask on the struggling boy's face. When he was finally anesthetized and still, the needle could be inserted.

Learning of this distressing circumstance, my anesthetic colleague suggested a different approach. Approaching the boy gently, he built some rapport and then asked the boy a question.

'In your living room at home, is there a light in the ceiling?' The boy nodded.

'How do you make the light work?' asked the doctor.

'You use the switch on the wall,' responded the boy.

'So how does that work? How does the switch make the light work?' The boy looked puzzled.

The doctor explained, 'How it works, there is a wire from the switch to the light. So when you flip the switch, it sends a signal to the light, to tell the light to go on.' The boy nodded his understanding.

The doctor asked the boy a strange question, 'If you look inside the wall, do you think you can tell me what color the wire is?'

The boy screwed up his eyes for a moment and then said, 'Yes, it's a red one!'

In turn, this kindly anesthesiologist asked the boy about the light, switch and wire in different rooms in his home. For each room, the boy told him the color of the wire. The doctor was full of praise and encouragement.

He asked a new question: 'Did you know that you can turn your arms and legs off?' The boy nodded.

'See if you can find the wire to your left leg and tell me what color it is.' The boy screwed up his eyes again and then nodding, told the doctor it was a green one.

'Do you think if you looked really hard you might be able to find the switch to turn your leg on and off?' Soon the boy nodded the affirmative.

'OK, now I'd like you to turn your left leg off. Tell me when it's done.'

When the doctor asked the boy to lift his right leg off the bed, it moved easily. The left leg wouldn't move at all.

'Why can't you move your left leg?' asked the doctor.

'Because it's turned off,' said the boy, in a matter-of-fact manner.

The doctor and boy continued to play the game, turning off and on the different arms and legs.

When the boy's left arm was turned off, the doctor said, 'If your arm is turned off, you won't be able to feel me touching your hand.' The boy nodded agreement.

'Can you feel this?' said the doctor, tapping him in the back of the hand. The boy shook his head.

'So if you can't feel your hand, I can put a needle in and you won't be able to feel it. Is it OK if I go ahead and do that now?' The boy nodded his assent, quite unperturbed at the suggestion.

When the doctor finished the procedure, he told the boy, 'OK. Now you can turn your arm on again.'

The whole procedure took about five minutes. Seeing this miracle of compassionate care, the boy's mother hugged the doctor and wept in his arms. The monthly hospital visits were no longer an ordeal.

This amazing doctor didn't hypnotize the boy; he merely employed suggestion.

It was an incredibly vivid demonstration of how the compassionate and mindful intention of a doctor can influence the physiology of a patient and turn trauma into healing.

Neuroscience says we can no longer uphold clinical detachment as a desirable or even realistic mode of relating to patients

Advances in neuroscience mean that we can no longer uphold clinical detachment as a desirable or even realistic mode of relating to patients. Detachment can strike into the hearts of our vulnerable patients, conveying an attitude of cold indifference.

As a psychological defense mechanism, to protect us from the suffering and tragedy we witness in the course of our work, it's shown to be deeply flawed.

Fortunately, the growing understanding of the pathways underlying our emotional responses, and the recent advances in positive psychology, allow us to appreciate that a deeply humanistic approach to the care of patients is the one that ultimately benefits us as much as our patients.

Chapter 9

MAKING TIME TO CARE

The angry and tearful family doctor challenged me directly: 'Get real, Robin! You have no understanding of the pressure we're under! I have to see a patient every ten to fifteen minutes and I can't possibly meet all their demands. The paperwork takes all my evening when I should be home with my children. I don't know how you can stand there saying that we have time to be more compassionate with patients!'

She sat down suddenly, fighting back floods of tears. It was an awkward moment in the middle of a workshop on compassionate caring. I stood on the stage while the audience wondered how I would react to this angry confrontation.

Get real! You have no understanding of the pressure we're under!

While doing my best to empathize with her distress, as a hospital specialist, I had no hope of relating to the reality of her practice setting out in the community. I was sure my answer would have no credibility for her. But I trusted to the wisdom of the audience and asked if there was anyone who could help respond to this situation.

Another family doctor stood up and offered to comment. She was similar in age and confessed that she, too, had struggled to manage the conflict between her busy clinical practice and childcare. There the similarity ended.

This doctor smiled warmly and radiated a calm and positive energy. 'I used to have a practice just like yours,' she indicated to the distressed doctor, 'but I found a way to reorganize my work so that I could care better for my patients and not be rushed all the time.'

Her solution was simple although it took some courage to implement the changes.

She realized the fundamental problem was that she was always practicing in a reactive mode, trying in a rush to solve all the urgent problems brought to her by patients. She often had an uneasy feeling that she wasn't getting to the heart of her patients' problems and certainly didn't have time to listen properly.

The solution was to restructure her appointment schedule so she could offer some 30-minute and 60-minute appointments and not fill the whole day with hurried 10 or 15-minute consultations.

As she began to explain her strategy, the angry doctor interrupted her saying, 'But you can't do that, you'll just lose income because you only get paid a fixed subsidy for each patient visit – it doesn't matter how long you see them!'

'Yes, you're right,' she acknowledged, 'I did lose some money in the beginning. But my patients really appreciated having the opportunity for an in-depth consultation and they were willing to pay an extra fee. Plus it gave us the opportunity to make a much better plan for future care, and build greater trust, so now we often just need a quick catch-up appointment.

'I now have more patients in my practice but I still have the flexibility to give them the time they need. If a patient comes with a lot of problems, we just book a longer session a few days later.

'It's really taken the pressure off and I enjoy my work so much more. I'd be really happy to help you explore ways you could make your own practice more flexible.'

At the end of the workshop I was gratified to see the two doctors walking away together, arm in arm. Healing often begins in a moment of connection, found in crisis.

A pressured healthcare system

'No-time-to-care' is a very widespread problem. A survey of 12,000 physicians in the USA showed that two-thirds of doctors often didn't have time to fully communicate and treat all patients [1].

Jill Maben, who we met in chapter 1 *Burnout*, found an institutional culture reinforcing a sense of busyness and intense work pressure in her research on the working lives of nurses in the United Kingdom [2]. The hurried physical care meant that nurses didn't have the time to attend to their patients' emotional needs.

And when I have polled health professionals in my networks about the biggest barrier to compassionate caring, the most frequent response is, "We don't have time to care."

When immersed in pressured practice, in the clinic, on a busy ward, or in the battleground of an emergency department, it can seem that demand is overwhelming. Very often, staffing shortage compounds the situation.

Having no time to care is the daily experience of very many health workers. When you're stuck in that hole, it's hard to see how things could be better without a major injection of new resources – an unlikely circumstance in today's under-funded healthcare system.

It's a major cause of dissatisfaction among practitioners: "Doctors' anguish seems to come from violating every day what they know they ought to be doing," said Renee Fox, a noted medical sociologist at the University of Pennsylvania [3]. "The pain is from the degree to which they still espouse values but can't live up to them."

And patients suffer too, when care gets pressured. In a critical review of hundreds of research papers examining empathy in clinical practice, the author noted, "Quite a few studies that indicate a relationship between being pressed for time and lowered empathy" [4].

Here's some ideas

Fortunately there are many inspiring examples of health workers who have overcome these difficulties and there's plenty of published research evidence to back up their claims. Here are the key strategies for making time to care:

- Investing a little time at the beginning of each patient contact to build trust and rapport. A minute or two spent here can save a great deal of wasted time later

- Using skills to get to the heart of the patient's concerns very quickly can eliminate those heart-sink moments when the patient brings up their real concern only at the end of a consultation - which must be started all over again!

- Practicing compassionate caring in parallel with necessary clinical tasks – both can be done at the same time

- Remembering that compassion is shown in the tiniest of acts – like the wonderful nurse who stopped to lift each wheel of the patient gurney over the bump in the floor, when transporting a patient with painfully unstable fractures

- Appreciating that the deepest and most meaningful connection with a patient occurs in a mere moment. Time stops when you are fully present

- Reorganizing care so that it is proactive, seeking to understand patient needs first, rather than always reacting to urgent new demands and becoming disorganized

- Critically examining care to eliminate many wasteful activities that add no value

- Reorganizing the workplace layout, flows and processes to make clinical tasks more efficient – the basis of many 'releasing time to care' projects

- Learning that compassionate care is more efficient in the long run. The reduction in patient complications, such as falls and pressure sores, lessens the workload

Disordered complexity

In a complex endeavor such as healthcare, systems tend to evolve over time without being explicitly designed for efficiency, or even effectiveness. We just keep adding layers and layers of activity on top of historical models of organization.

A good analogy is the design of Web Browsers for surfing the Internet. The latest version of Internet Explorer (IE9) from Microsoft requires a 27MB download, according to download.cnet.com.

By contrast, Chrome, the widely admired and popular browser from Google has a download file of only 0.6MB.

Both browsers fulfill the same function yet the Microsoft product uses nearly fifty times as much code to get the same end result.

The difference is that Google started from scratch and designed a highly efficient and speedy browser using completely new code.

Microsoft, on the other hand, is often developing products on top of a shaky foundation of bug-ridden historical code, full of layered complexity. Every time they find a problem, they have to put a new sticking plaster on it and ask you to download yet another 'update'.

If I put my engineering hat on and examine the work processes I observe on a typical hospital ward, I find a huge amount of activity that is wasteful, disorganized, repetitive, or achieves no useful purpose at all.

For instance, it's commonplace to find a model of care where the 'medical team' ultimately responsible for the safe care of patients have 'their' patients scattered in many locations across different hospital wards. So the essential coordination of care – between the doctors, who are organized in hospital-wide 'teams', and the ward-based nurses and therapist – breaks down.

This fragmented care and lack of information sharing is readily apparent to the patient, who quickly gets used to multiple members of the care 'team' asking the same questions, over and over, duplicating the written records.

An enormous amount of health workers' precious time is wasted making phone calls or walking from one end of the hospital to another.

If the medical and nursing teams were co-located in a single ward, the communication and coordination of care would be enhanced and time could be liberated for compassionate patient care.

Our physical work environments are also often poorly designed for purpose. The typical medication room, equipment store, and clinical supply room of a ward are fully of chaotic processes, like six chefs who are all trying to work at once in a poorly designed kitchen!

Releasing time to care with redesign

Often the workflows can be dramatically enhanced by a simple reorganization of storage, and standardization of common clinical tasks. We don't need to rebuild the hospital to make many gains and the increase in efficiency can be startling.

The UK's National Health Service (NHS) has found ways to eliminate much of the layered complexity and poor organization in a typical workplace [5]. The Releasing Time to Care project:

- increased the time spent on direct care by 20%
- cut nurse handover time by a third
- reduced medicine round time by 63%
- cut meal wastage rates from 7% to 1%

The Director of Nursing commented it was a program that, at face value, seemed relatively simple and straightforward, yet generated huge benefits for individual nurses, patients and the organization. One only has to visit a ward where some of the modules have been implemented to see the difference.

"The ward usually appeared calm – however busy. There was a place for all equipment so it was less cluttered, cupboards were tidy and only contained what was actually needed; vital observations were recorded, there are less patient falls, reduced drug errors and above all, happier patients and staff.

"Ward teams appeared to work and act as a cohesive body, working for the greater good of the patients they cared for. Waste was eliminated allowing more time to spend in direct care with patients. This supported nurses to do 'what they came into nursing to do'."

The same methodology used in Scotland resulted in direct patient care time increasing between 13% and 43% across five pilot sites [6]. Both the English and Scottish programs reported improvement in patient safety, patient satisfaction, and reduced costs.

The researchers explained how they adopted the 'lean' methodology pioneered by Taiichi Ohino, a Production Engineer at Toyota Car Production in the 1950's [5].

In essence, Ohino found that staff and resources were often undertaking activities that provided no benefit. Toyota staff were trained and encouraged to spot any wasteful or unproductive processes.

More importantly, once spotted, staff were empowered to eliminate them. This process was referred to as the 'Respect for Humanity System' as it was felt that any waste squanders scarce resources.

But what can I do?

It seems there's little 'respect for humanity' in many healthcare workplaces and it's easy to feel helpless about changing your own work conditions. After all, the 'releasing time to care' projects were national programs, well resourced and supported by senior leaders.

What can individuals do? A great deal, as it turns out.

Most of the strategies for making-time-to-care at the beginning of this chapter are personal choices and habits of practice. As an individual you may not be able to redesign your workplace but you can change the way you relate to patients and work colleagues. You don't need permission from your boss, or even approval from your peers.

The examples from the 'releasing time to care project' show the possibility of change. Imagine how your practice could change if you had 20% to 40% more time for direct patient care during a shift?

At one of the Scottish pilot sites, the change in staff morale was remarkable. Before the pilot, 75% of staff described staff morale as 'rotten'. Three months later, 78% of the staff said staff morale was 'brilliant' [6].

These disordered workplaces provide a vivid metaphor for what is going on in our own minds when care has become over-busy and stressed. The hospital wards were cluttered, disorganized, full of constant interruptions, and contained many activities that added no value to patient care. To make time to care, it is necessary to restore some calm and stillness in our minds.

Care arises with personal presence. The only way to be 'present' is to be fully aware in the present moment. You can't be present when ruminating angrily about the past or fretting about the future.

When we make time to slow down, we become more effective. Time expands and precious moments fill the space we create.

In 2009, I was invited to give a speech to a prestigious health policy forum in London.

Some of the most influential health leaders were in the room, attending by personal invitation – it was an exclusive event. As the keynote speaker for the event, I had spent hours carefully crafting my speech for a 40 minute slot. Twelve hours before the event, I learned that the allocated time for my speech was only twenty minutes!

My initial panic gave way to a more useful thought: If I have so little time to talk, I had better slow down. Rather than filling my speech with so many ideas and stories, I realized I had to get to the heart of the matter and make sure I really connected with my audience.

The best speakers know this. They always put periods of silence in their speeches and bring the room to a point of still reflection.

So the first step in finding time to care is simply to stop. Give your patient complete attention. Bring stillness to your mind and be attentive to what is happening. Magic happens in these precious moments.

> **The first step in finding time to care is simply to stop. Give your patient complete attention**

In our clockwork analogy of the Universe, we have an idea of time as something rigid, punctuated and inflexible. This sense of time is reinforced when our care becomes nothing more than a series of tasks. When care is mechanical, time becomes rigid.

But the human experience of time is quite different. In moments of close connection, time stands still. Research shows that patients who attend a doctor skilled in interpersonal connection believe their appointment was much longer than the allocated time.

So even though the patients might have spent only fifteen minutes with the doctor, they feel as if they spent much longer. They say, 'The doctor gave me all the time I needed. She really listened to all my concerns.'

Analysis of videotaped doctor-patient consultations showed that those consultations where the doctor picked up patient cues were actually shorter than those where the doctor failed to notice or respond [7]. So although the consultation is interrupted by the patient's signals, the overall result is quicker and more satisfying for both parties.

Magic occurs in moments, which is why our language is full of this idea. 'Moment' means both an instant in time and also an event of great significance. So we speak of 'an event of great moment' and of 'momentous events'.

The word 'moment' also has a meaning in physics to do with the force of a spinning object. This accords with our idea of momentous events being 'turning points' in history.

Healing occurs when you open up a sacred space between practitioner and patient. You need to be deliberate in creating the conditions for this deep connection.

Like it or not, the way we behave as health practitioners profoundly affects our patients within seconds of meeting. When we bring an attitude of busyness and hurry into our interaction with patients, we shut out caring and compassion. Patients sense this within seconds. The unspoken message from the health worker is, 'Don't bother me, don't ask questions, don't make demands – I'm too busy and important for your petty concerns.'

So the attitude and beliefs we carry about time pressure profoundly affect our patient caring.

Even in the busiest care settings, there are some practitioners who move through the day with unhurried grace. They get much more done than their busy and stressed colleagues – and have a lot more fun and satisfaction in a day's work.

Slowing down, making the connection, and opening up the space of healing requires both an attitudinal shift and learning new skills.

Seven practices

Here are seven simple practices you can follow to ensure you always have time to care for your patients:

1. Collect yourself before you meet your next patient

Collecting yourself literally means, pulling together the pieces. When over-busy, our attention becomes fragmented among competing demands. Pause, take a breath and think about your attitude. Are you going to bring softness, kindness and openhearted compassion into the room or else project an attitude of ill humor and busyness? It's amazing how many health workers are grumpy with their patients.

2. Be aware of your body language

The stressed health worker will march into the patient's room all grim faced and taut – lips compressed, no smile, no eye contact, no greeting, firing off questions or instructions. Be the opposite. Smile with the genuine pleasure of meeting another person and the opportunity of an intimate connection. Keep your body language open and soft. Don't cross your arms. Make eye contact. Offer a touch.

3. Make introductions

During a hospital stay, the average patient will probably meet fifty or more health workers. Many don't bother to introduce themselves. The typical security/ID badge is worn on the belt, invisible to the patient. So take care with introductions. Don't just give your name but explain your role. If there are other people in the room, find out how they are related to the patient. Greet them as potential team members. Ask the patient how he or she would like to be addressed. Some prefer a first name, some a more formal address.

4. Tell patients you have time

In the Studer Group work on hourly patient rounds, nurses were trained to use words that trigger patient needs [8]. At the conclusion of the round, nurses are instructed to say to every patient, 'Is there anything else I can do for you before I leave? I have time.'

The addition of those three words, 'I have time,' significantly increases the number of patients who responded with a request. Most patients know that health professionals are very busy. They don't like to bother their caregiver so important things are often left unsaid.

Telling patients you have time becomes a self-fulfilling prophecy. It's a good habit.

5. Be sensitive to the power relationship, show respect

Patients are at a profound disadvantage. They find themselves in a strange and frightening environment, they are often robbed of clothing and identity, they are afraid about the consequences of their illness, and they may be hungry, cold and sleep deprived.

All these factors reinforce the role of patients as passive and helpless participants in their care.

And what do groups of health professionals typically do on a ward round? They crowd around the bed standing over the patient.

So you have to work hard to overcome this disadvantage. Get down to the level of the patient so that you are talking eye to eye. Often there's no chair next to the patient's bed so I either crouch or kneel on the floor, or ask permission to sit on the bed.

I observe some doctors who ask if they can sit on the bed and then plonk themselves down before the patient has a chance to respond! So show respect. Really ask permission. Don't sit down until the patient has approved.

We are so familiar with all the rituals and tasks of care that we often forget they represent a grave intrusion on the privacy and dignity of the patient. In ordinary society it's not acceptable to touch strangers except in certain ritualized ways, like a handshake. Measuring blood pressure is an intrusion. We don't ordinarily have permission to remove clothing, wrap a cuff tight around the arm, inflate it to painful pressure levels, or stand so close when making observations.

Part of opening up the space for trust and healing is being deeply respectful. Ask permission for each task in patient care, whether it's to measure the blood pressure, take the temperature, listen to the chest or give an injection.

6. Let the patient set the agenda

I've always been a friendly and courteous doctor. What I didn't realise for most of my career was that I resolutely set the agenda for every patient encounter. As a hospital specialist, my source of identity and self-esteem arose from being an expert. I took my job and myself rather seriously.

Roles are very powerful in shaping behavior. I had no idea how intimidating I was as a medical specialist seeing patients in my consulting room. I would greet my patients with a smile, make quick introductions and then launch immediately into the clinical subject: 'Mrs Jones I see you are coming for a gall bladder operation next week. Tell me about your asthma.'

At the end of each consultation I would ask the patient if she had any questions. The answer was always, 'No.' Feeling satisfied with doing a good job, I'd move on to the next patient.

Over the years, I developed a little more empathy. I began to sense that patients might have hidden concerns. I modified my closing question to, 'Is there anything you want to ask me or anything you're worried about?'

One day I was astonished by the response. The patient was a twenty-eight year old professional woman attending surgery to have four impacted wisdom teeth removed under general anesthesia. She was obviously intelligent and well educated. I asked about her experience of surgery and anesthesia and did she have any problems or bad reactions to the anesthetic. She said, 'No.'

But when I asked my concluding question she began to weep silently. With much hesitation she then told me a horrifying story.

Three years before, she had a general anesthetic for abdominal surgery. Half way through the operation the anesthetic wore off and she woke up when the surgery was still continuing. She was completely paralyzed and unable to move. She could feel the pain of the surgery and hear the voices of the surgeons. Her eyes were taped closed. She had no way of signaling her terror.

This experience was so deeply traumatizing that she discharged herself early from hospital and told nobody what had happened. She had suffered nightmares for years and had many other symptoms of a post-traumatic stress disorder. I was the first health professional she had ever told.

I was deeply shocked by her story. Unintended awareness during general anesthesia is a very rare complication. In twenty-five years of practice I have come across only a few cases and none so disturbing.

But what shocked me equally is that under direct questioning, this intelligent and assured professional had denied any previous problems with anesthesia.

Over time I have come to understand that the more frightened a patient is, the less likely they will confess their fears. Some patients will even withhold information critical for their safe care. Many patients will endure surgery or medical treatment that they didn't want – simply because they go along with all the health professionals who provide care without ever stopping to ask what's important for the patient.

Over time I have come to understand that the more frightened a patient is, the less likely they will confess their fears

So now I have changed my practice. I pay more careful attention to introductions and building rapport. I explain my role and try to put the patient at ease. I greet the patient as a fellow human being and try to learn something about their ordinary lives – just the smallest thing makes a difference. I explain the process of care and ask the patient if that's OK?

Then I say, 'Before we start it would be really helpful for me to know what's on your mind. Is there some question or thought that keeps going round in your head?'

It's amazing how often this question saves time:

1. You discover patients who didn't need or want the treatment. They are so happy when someone actually listens to them for the first time!

2. You find out that patients have already come to the conclusion you were going to spend an hour persuading them to accept.

3. You uncover the clue that provides a critical element in diagnosis and treatment.

4. You avoid unanticipated complications.

5. You put to rest fears and anxieties so the patients' healing and recovery will be quicker.

6. You don't waste a whole hour talking about peripheral subjects only to have the patient at the door confessing that there was something else important to discuss.

7. Gentle humor

Many studies show that fun and laughter have the power to heal. A colleague of mine, Dr Peter Spitzer, is the founder and medical director of a national network of clown doctors in Australia [9]. His most recent work in residential care centers for the elderly suggests that you can begin to reverse the process of dementia through clowning, fun and laughter [10, 11].

Gentle humor is a great way to help put people at ease, build rapport, and have more fun at work.

I've just returned from a mercy mission to repatriate a dear friend dying of motor neuron disease. Derek normally lives in New Zealand but in desperation had sought specialist medical care in Germany, leaving behind his wife and young son.

There is no established cure or treatment for motor neuron disease and our poor friend found himself stranded with no money and unable to travel. Derek was almost paralyzed and unable to speak. Drinking and eating were very difficult. The journey back home was an agonizing thirty-six hours of air travel. My wife and I flew from New Zealand to Germany and back in four days, so we could nurse Derek on the return journey.

Derek is a brilliant man trapped in a ruined body. He can smile and cry. The only other communication was by means of letters painfully inscribed on a writing tablet, often too distorted to decipher. It might take ten or fifteen minutes of painful trial and error to discover simply that his pillow needed adjusting. We had to attend to his every need and watch over him each minute of the long journey home.

We had a brief respite at Dubai airport and after pleading with airline staff we managed to get Derek into the first class lounge where he could lie down on a sofa. We finally got him comfortable and took photographs of the grinning Derek in the lounge. Sensing a lightening of the mood I knelt at his side, put my palms together in supplication, and bowing my head said, 'Master, your every wish is my command!'

We all ended up in hysterics of laughter. It was a magical moment in a journey of unendurable suffering.

When we are caught up in laughter, time stops and suffering is banished. It's an instant cure for many ills. Many of the things we do in the course of healthcare are bizarre and ridiculous. There's so much potential for fun and laughter even with dying patients.

For the best reminder of the role of laughter in medicine, watch the movie Patch Adams (1998). Robin Williams gives an exuberant performance in the role of the real-life Dr Patch Adams, founder of the Gesundheit Institute, which is dedicated to bring fun, laughter, humanity and healing to the practice of healthcare [12].

A whole-system approach to making time to care

The very best results come from putting together all these strategies into a whole-system approach for humanizing care. The best example I have found is at Inova Health System in northern Virginia where the leaders integrated a human caring model into professional nursing practice across four hospitals [13].

I detailed many of their practices in chapter 2, *Kindness*.

They found that listening, providing information, encouraging expressions of concern, and helping cope with difficult situations actually took no additional time. But the leaders also included a relentless focus on improving work processes and freeing up time to care.

Phase 1 of their integrated program was a deliberate focus on decreasing work intensity by eliminating wasteful processes.

For instance they piloted use of an admission nurse, whose sole job was to admit, discharge and transfer patients on the medical unit. This initiative reduced the average time to admit a patient from 76 minutes to 56 minutes; resulting in a 20-minute decrease in time for each patient admission.

They also introduced a "VoiceCare" system, a telephone voicemail system for report, allowing for prerecorded patient history to be repeated each shift.

VoiceCare expedited shift change communication by 3.6 minutes per patient per report, saving more than an hour of nurses' time on a typical 20-bed ward.

Phase 2 of the program was creating a human caring environment, using the freed up time to reinvest in direct patient care. The objective was to improve staff nurse satisfaction and reduce turnover rates by developing the art of nursing in a caring and healing environment, within an acute care setting.

Nurse's work satisfaction scores improved, as did scores for teamwork and mutual support. The workplace that facilitates compassionate patient care is a great place to work. One study participant said:

"I have been a nurse about 2 years now, and I had been feeling frustrated because I was not able to spend enough time interacting with my patients. I was actually thinking of leaving nursing because I was so discouraged.

By being able to have the time to implement the human caring interventions, my perspective has changed and I have the support from my coworkers and nursing leadership to spend time with my patients. It has made all the difference for me, and I cannot imagine being anything but a nurse."

Chapter 10

BUILDING A BETTER SYSTEM

Fifty community leaders were gathered to collaborate on a project to keep our young people safe in the community.

Too many of our teens were killed or injured in car crashes, violent assaults, by suicide, drowning, fire, or overdoses of drugs or alcohol.

It wasn't the easiest group to facilitate. These were people accustomed to authority: the Chief of Police; the Chair of the Health Board; the Chief Fire Officer; City Counselors; business executives; school principals, church leaders and tribal chiefs.

When the time came for decisions on project structure and allocation of resources, the arguments began. Who was going to be in charge?

At this moment of confrontation, we heard the quiet voice of Peter Senge, an internationally renowned thought leader in the principles of organizational learning, building community and sustainable solutions [1]. He'd generously agreed to help facilitate the meeting.

'Look at the rain forest,' he said, indicating the spectacular mountain views from the windows of the conference center.

'There's a system of infinite complexity and interdependence and yet nobody is in charge. We don't always need authority systems to do good work together.'

In our work to re-humanize healthcare, we'd do well to take nature's example. The rain forest that Senge indicated is a system in perfect health, an eco-system in perfect balance, endlessly sustained. Each plant flourishes in its own niche, gaining all the nourishment and shelter it needs.

A degraded ecosystem

When European settlers came to New Zealand in the 1800's they found much of the land covered in forest. To build farms they first felled and burned the trees, converting forest into pasture. This was the fate of Tiritiri Matangi Island. Just four kilometers off the mainland, the island became a sheep farm and also the site of a lighthouse that helped guide ships into Auckland.

Aerial photographs of the 220-hectare island in the 1960's show the land quite bare, devoid of trees except for small gullies and rocky cliffs where vestiges of native forest survived. Birdsong was lost with the forest. The island was windswept and silent save for the scuttling of rats and other introduced pests.

In many areas of New Zealand the forest has fallen silent because of the devastating impact of introduced species. Possums destroy the forest canopy and prevent the trees from flowering. Rats, stoats, cats and possums prey on birds' nests, stealing eggs and killing the fledglings. The bird populations have declined or vanished.

Today, Tiritiri Matangi Island is a scientific reserve, sixty percent re-forested and showcasing a profusion of birdlife unknown in mainland New Zealand [2].

The birds have no natural predators and are unafraid of humans. As you walk along the many miles of paths, the birds flock around and the air is rich with birdsong.

The island is an important conservation reserve and is home to many endangered species, including the Takahe, one of the rarest birds in the world, and the Tuatara, a prehistoric lizard.

I began to think about healthcare as an ecosystem after a visit to this inspirational wildlife sanctuary, which is just an hour by ferry from the waterfront in downtown Auckland.

Most of birds on the island were not artificially introduced – they simply arrived, flourished in the enriched environment, and multiplied. When the ecosystem is restored, the flowers bloom and birdsong is heard again. Here is a profound lesson for our work on restoring a caring and compassionate healthcare system.

Here are some of the success factors at Tiritiri Matangi:

1. The efforts are contained within a geographically defined area – in this case a small island.

2. Predators and pests were eliminated with an intensive trapping and eradication program.

3. Strict bio-security at the boundary prevents the accidental re-introduction of pests, such as rats or noxious weeds.

4. The process of environmental restoration began with the planting of 300,000 trees over a ten years period.

5. The saplings were grown from seeds harvested from remaining forest on the island. The 'eco-sourced' seedlings were nurtured until big enough to be planted in the wild.

6. A huge community of volunteers - today numbering 1,300 - does almost all of the work. This closely knit community has a powerfully shared purpose and vision.

7. The results of the volunteers' hard work are highly visible. Each year more of the island was replanted, the trees grew, the birds multiplied, the flowers and fruits of the forest bloomed and ripened, and the birdsong grew ever louder.

8. As the birds returned in large numbers, the forest began to re-multiply with a greater diversity of species and richness of habitat. The birds spreading seeds and fruits are an essential part of the process of natural regeneration.

9. Volunteers created many miles of trails around the island so visitors can appreciate the rich diversity of habitat, find the many different bird species, and enjoy the natural beauty.

10. Scientific research and an intensive education program back the whole restoration project. School children and other visitors learn about the project in an education center, manned by volunteers.

Healthcare also has a natural ecosystem – of kindness, caring and compassion – but it too has become severely degraded. Too much of human caring has been replaced by technology, tasks and procedures. We create sterile, clinical environments rather than natural places of healing. And we don't take care of our young and our vulnerable.

Creating a 'conservation island' for compassionate caring

When we build on the inspiration of Tiritiri Matangi Island, it suggests some clear strategies for restoring compassion and caring in our workplace.

1. Create a 'conservation' area

We can learn from the success of the Tiritiri Matangi Island project. If we want to re-humanize healthcare and to restore caring and compassion perhaps we can begin with small conservation areas where we make intensive efforts to restore the caring ecosystem?

To restore the natural eco-system of kindness, caring and compassion, many different elements need to be addressed. It's hard to do this in a large institution – better to start a pilot program in a circumscribed physical area, like one ward or department.

Make sure you define the boundaries.

2. Eliminating the 'pests' that destroy the eco-system

There is an expression in healthcare: 'We eat our young'. It's a rueful admission that young, vulnerable students and newly qualified health workers are bullied, abused and sometimes spat out of the system, never to return. There is little sense of nurturing, protection or allowing our young to develop as healthy, resilient and caring professionals.

When we set aside an area – maybe a ward or clinic – the first step is to eliminate pests and put in place the bio-security. What do I mean by pests? The bullying, abuse, discrimination and even tantrums that are so widespread in healthcare:

High rates of bullying are reported in surveys including 44% of community nurses [3], 50% of junior doctors [4], and 25% of postgraduate hospital dentists [5]. A larger percentage of health workers report witnessing the bullying of others.

A follow-up study of 2154 newly graduated health workers in Denmark showed a strong relationship between exposure to bullying and workers quitting their jobs [6]. Those who left their jobs complained of poor leadership, being exposed to negative behavior and health problems.

Disruptive behavior by physicians is a persistent threat to patient safety. An Institute of Safe Medication Practices survey showed that 49% of health practitioners have felt pressured by bullies to dispense or administer a drug despite serious and unresolved safety concerns, and 40% have kept quiet rather than question a known intimidator [7].

Other quoted studies have shown that victims learn to cope by avoiding the abuser, even if this means failing to call for advice and avoiding making suggestions that might improve care.

A very large survey of fifty Veterans Hospital Administration (VHA) hospitals in the USA showed that bullying had negative effects on both nurses and physicians, on stress, frustration, concentration, communication, collaboration, information transfer, and workplace relationships [8].

Most respondents believed those effects led onto medical errors, which impacted on patient safety, patient mortality, the quality of care, and patient satisfaction.

There are few studies of the emotional impact that bullying health workers have on vulnerable patients. One survey reported that 46% of nurses and 30% of physicians had seen health professionals berating patients [9].

I have seen an obstetrician and a midwife furiously argue across the bed of a frightened women in advanced labor. When your very life depends on the collaboration, teamwork and good judgment of health professionals, the sight of those professionals losing control can only be terrifying.

When health workers are stressed, angry, and frustrated then compassion and caring are the first casualties.

While I strongly advocate an appreciative inquiry approach to all other aspects of strengthening caring and compassion, the impact of bullying is so pernicious that a systematic strategy of 'pest control' is necessary.

Just as rats, stoats and other predators prey on the weak and vulnerable, bullying in healthcare does most damage to our students, young professionals and the vulnerable patients in our care.

This behavior is so commonplace it has become normalized and invisible. An important strategy in dealing with bullying is for leaders to name the behaviors that are not tolerated: physical abuse, condescension, insults, disrespect, abusive anger, berating colleagues or patients, yelling/raising the voice, and abusive language.

What can you do? The problem is more easily fixed than you think. In practical experience, about 80% of those who intimidate or cause distress to others are completely unaware of this negative impact of their behavior. One or two instances of constructive feedback will resolve the problem.

These are good-hearted people who want to do their best. They are often shocked and embarrassed to discover that their behavior caused problems for others. Because they lack insight, you have to explicitly describe the kinds of behavior that cause problems and the impact it has on others.

The next 15% need a bit more work. I have personally coached physicians who show disruptive behavior and often a problem can be resolved with two or three 15-minute sessions of coaching and support.

We need to be compassionate to those who show difficult behavior because it's often a marker of personal stress or health problems.

The final 5% of persistently disruptive health workers need to be managed in a disciplinary framework that offers coaching and support but also spells out potential consequences including dismissal.

In these days of health worker shortages, when it can be so difficult to recruit nurses, therapists or physicians to fill gaps in the roster, it's commonplace for leaders to tolerate bad behavior. This is a serious error. Happy hospitals don't have trouble attracting and retaining staff. For every disruptive worker expelled from the organization, ten more will queue at the door saying, 'I want to work there!'

We tend to think people's behavior is largely driven by innate factors like personality so we tend to greatly underestimate the influence of context or situation. Most bullies are cowards. When you stand up to them, they back off pretty quickly.

One day in the emergency department I witnessed the chairman of a medical department, a very senior and physically intimidating man, yelling at an ER doctor. Before I could do anything, the charge nurse, a tiny person barely five feet tall, intervened masterfully.

She took the elbow of the yelling doctor and wordlessly led him across to the opposite corner of the room. Gazing up at his face, she gently said, 'Doctor, I'm sorry, but that behavior is not acceptable in our department.' He immediately apologized and made amends with his ER colleague.

When we use compassion and gentleness we can disarm even the most senior and aggressive members of staff. If the rules are explicit and there is zero tolerance for disruptive behavior, then people quickly learn to modulate their words and actions. You just need to define the boundaries of your 'compassion island' and practice bio-security. No pests allowed in here.

3. Collecting the 'seeds of caring' through appreciative inquiry

Having eliminated the pests and protected the young and vulnerable, it's time to start restoring the caring eco-system.

On Tiritiri Matangi Island, they re-populated the forest by collecting seeds from the few remaining trees and cultivating the native seedlings in greenhouses - so-called eco-sourcing. How do we do this in healthcare?

The answer is everything we need is already present, just like on the island.

Health workers come into the professional with a deep desire to care for patients. Even in the most degraded work environment, there are instances of wonderful kindness, care and compassion. The way to find these seeds of caring is to use appreciative inquiry. This will be explored further in chapter 11, *Compassionate Leadership*.

Instead of focusing on problems, all of the staff members can be brought together in a process that asks questions about peak experiences in compassionate caring, times when health workers felt most connected to the work they do. Inspiring stories emerge. People discover unsuspected strengths.

The authors of *Appreciative Inquiry in Healthcare* ask [10]:

- Tell us about a time when all of the pieces fell into place and you and your team were able to deliver exceptional care to a patient?

- Describe an interaction with a patient when you were able to make time stand still, forget about your other obligations, and be completely in the moment.

- Over the course of your career, you have encountered many patients. If you could pick one patient who stands out because of his or her story, who would that person be?

- Talk about the last time a patient thanked you for listening. What prompted you to listen? What did you do or say that allowed the patient or family to ask the right questions at the right time?

The application of appreciative inquiry goes far beyond patient care. It's equally important in fostering the conditions for working together in teams, caring for the caregivers, experiencing the awe and wonder of our jobs, hiring and keeping the best employees, creating a positive atmosphere, and fostering patient safety.

I know of no other process that is so successful in engaging every single member of the healthcare team: therapists, clerks, nurses, physicians, care assistants, porters, technicians, cleaners, receptionists, team leaders – everyone has a role to play in compassionate caring.

And when shared purpose is developed through stories of extraordinary teamwork and collaboration, morale is dramatically enhanced and the working atmosphere becomes positive and inviting.

Like the birdsong in the restored forest, the smiles, contentment, and expressions of kindness and appreciation are apparent to all visitors. This is a place that will attract and retain like-minded health workers.

4. Support nurturing leadership styles

You'll recall that I started this chapter with an observation by Peter Senge that the perfectly self-organizing rain forest didn't need anyone to be in charge.

The volunteers on Tiritiri Matangi Island don't instruct the trees and birds; rather they create the conditions for them to flourish and live together in harmony.

Leadership styles in healthcare make a big difference to the work environment. Too often we witness transactional leadership focused solely on task completion, production targets, process measures, and budgets – as if healthcare was a factory, not a complex human endeavor.

Transformational and relational leadership styles are needed to enhance health worker satisfaction and create healthy work environments [11].

Studies that explore the relationship between organizational culture and quality improvement show that hospitals known to be good places to work have a lower Medicare mortality rate [12].

Furthermore, organizational support for staff is known to affect job satisfaction and burnout, which impact quality of care.

Blindly pursuing productivity and financial indicators creates self-perpetuating elements of culture than run counter to quality.

In a study of the organizational configuration of hospitals succeeding in attracting and retaining nurses, the attractive hospitals have many of the features of healthy workplaces, they're less hierarchical and benefit from high levels of trust between workers [13].

Low turnover hospitals in the study had no staffing vacancies but those with high turnover suffered vacancy rates as high as 15.8%.

"Attractive hospitals have a distinctive profile characterized by intentional, systematic and collaborative efforts to maximize employee well-being by providing well-designed and meaningful jobs, a supportive social organizational environment, and accessible and equitable opportunities for professional development and work-life enhancement."

Investing in the health and wellbeing of employees is shown to be a valuable investment in any business, according to a major research program for the UK government, conducted by PricewaterhouseCoopers and adopted by the British NHS [14].

"Programme costs can quickly be translated into financial benefits, either through cost savings or additional revenue generation, as a consequence of the improvement in a wide range of intermediate business measures."

Authentic leadership – genuine, trustworthy, reliable, compassionate, and believable – is crucial for the development of healthy work environments for nursing practice [15].

"Healthy work environments are supportive of the whole human being, are patient-focused, and are joyful workplaces. Authentic leaders develop heart and compassion by getting to know the life stories of those with whom they work and by engaging coworkers in shared meaning."

Importantly the link is made between authentic leadership and the findings of positive psychology. The leaders' generation of confidence, hope, optimism, resiliency and positive emotions facilitates the followers' positive attitudes, behaviors, and performance outcomes.

5. Create a 'nest of caring'

The bird nests on Titirangi Island are also a great analogy for caring. The vulnerable infant birds are provided food, warmth, and comfort – the things we most often fail to provide to patients stuck in hospital.

Large numbers of hospital patients are left starving, like the young woman lying on her back in spinal traction who could not see or reach the meal tray brought into her room. Too often the ward staff were too busy to ensure she was fed.

Sometimes it's organizational factors that cause hunger, like the patient waiting nil-by-mouth for emergency surgery that gets canceled day after day because of overbooking of acute cases.

Hypothermia is common among frail, elderly hospital patients. It dramatically increases the risk of complications and causes profound misery and a state of helplessness.

In 2010 I prolapsed a disc in my neck and suffered acute nerve compression. Following two days and a night in increasingly severe pain, no sleep, and nil-by-mouth status, it was the cold that finally defeated me.

After changing into a thin hospital gown in preparation for an MRI scan, I waited in a freezing room, shivering uncontrollably. I could hear voices next door but I was too miserable and helpless to even call out for a blanket. This was a hospital where I worked as a senior doctor but I had lost all my power.

Unrelieved pain is a common cause of patient complaints, particularly among those sitting for many hours in the waiting room of the Emergency Room. The drugs to relieve pain are readily available but there's no system to reliably supply them to suffering patients.

These three failings – the lack of food, warmth and comfort – are systematic problems rather than the failings of individuals. They arise particularly when there are budget and staffing shortages but the cost saving is false. Malnutrition, hypothermia and unrelieved pain dramatically increase complications, inhibit healing and prolong hospital stay.

We can't claim to have a compassionate healthcare system if we don't meet simple human needs like food, warmth and comfort.

So perhaps an idea is to call your island of compassion 'a nest of caring', which translates to *kohanga atawhai* in the Maori language of New Zealand.

6. Use volunteers

A close-knit community of volunteers did almost all the restoration work on Tiritiri Matangi Island. The ferry company offers free passage to volunteers and the day I visited, there was a large group of senior citizens on the boat.

From their warm greetings, enthusiasm and good humor it soon became apparent they were among the happy volunteers who had helped plant 300,000 trees.

In the developed world, with our huge healthcare budgets, we are accustomed to healthcare provided almost exclusively by paid professionals.

As a result we greatly neglect the potential contribution of patients, families and volunteers (including staff volunteering their time).

For an example of the abundance of resources that can be liberated when we think more flexibly, consider Cuba. According to the United Nations Statistics Division, this impoverished small nation has exactly the same life expectancy as the USA, and a lower infant mortality rate, 6 per 1,000 births, as against 8 per 1,000 births in the USA [16].

But Cuba spends on healthcare, per citizen, less than one twentieth of the amount in the USA, $300 per year compared with more than $7,000 in the USA [17].

We can learn a lot from the creativity of countries that have tackled major social and health problems when almost no money is available.

One of my heroes is Dr Vera Cordeiro, a pediatrician who has transformed health outcomes in the poorest parts of Brazil.

Her story, among many others, is written in a book, *How to Change the World – Social Entrepreneurs and the Power of New Ideas* [18].

Cordeiro founded Associação Saúde Criança Renascer (Rebirth: Association for Children's Health) while working on the pediatric ward at Hospital da Lagoa, a public hospital in Rio that served many of the poorest families living in the urban slums.

Cordeiro could not bear to see so many children discharged from hospital only to return sick again within a few weeks.

The illnesses she treated were the by-products of poverty and unsanitary living conditions in the favelas, the shanty towns that sprawl up the hillsides overlooking the richer parts of the city. Every day Cordeiro saw children with pneumonia, tuberculosis, rheumatic fever, anemia, birth defects, leptospirosis, and infected skin lesions.

These children received acute hospital treatment but were then discharged back into the community without support or follow-up. Cordeiro labeled the healthcare that ignored poverty and the conditions of the family as 'false treatment'.

Between 1991 and 1997, the new follow-up services created by Cordeiro led to a sixty percent drop in readmissions to Lagoa's pediatric unit. The impact according to the director of the unit was stunning.

Doctors and nurses were now able to do what they had trained to do: heal. By 2007, Cordeiro had extended her work to sixteen public hospitals in Rio de Janeiro, São Paulo and Recife.

Cordeira's association for children's health relies almost entirely on a volunteer workforce. Many other inspiring stories in the book about social entrepreneurs have the same theme. It's a lesson we need to take to heart in our work re-humanizing healthcare. Meeting basic needs like food, warmth and comfort does not require the application of highly trained health professionals.

Family members, healthcare students, high-school volunteers, and senior citizens can all play a major role in helping to meet the basic human needs of sick and vulnerable patients. Volunteering is a role for qualified health professionals too.

Most health professionals are highly constrained in their work environment – the sheer pressure of work, the unrelenting demand, and the restrictive rules of institutions limit their compassionate contribution. When you volunteer your time, you experience a sudden liberation: many of the rules don't apply any more.

When at boarding school in England – a hideous institution – I had nowhere to go for a half-term break. My family was overseas. While the teachers took their holiday break, a small groups of friends and I were left to run free in the school grounds with no rules. What delicious liberation! There was a certain amount of mischief making.

If you choose to attend your workplace outside of normal duties, there's a similar sense of liberation. Nobody is there to tell you how to spend your time, although of course you are bound by the usual professional ethics and organizational policies.

At the end of your shift, you might choose to sit quietly with a patient for half an hour, hold their hand, and really listen to their concerns. The tension and strains of the busy day will quickly melt away and you'll go home inspired with a new sense of purpose.

Here's some ideas of how you might volunteer your time:

Maybe you're concerned about the number of hospital patients leaving food untouched and want to document this problem?

Give up a little of your time one Saturday lunchtime and inspect the food trolleys as they come out of the wards. Take a camera. The photographs of multiple un-touched food trays will be a powerful image.

Befriend the porter who delivers and collects the trays – you'll be surprised how much he cares about the patients he meets. Maybe he's willing to do a simple data collection for you?

Or if patient comfort is a concern, recruit a student to do a simple study of the prevalence of patients in the ER waiting room who have severe, untreated pain.

All he needs is a simple analogue pain scale, a clipboard, and a piece of paper to record results. Given the computer skills of our young generations, you'll probably find he can create an iPhone application to automate the data collection! The results will motivate your colleagues to address this problem.

If hypothermia of elderly patients is a worry, talk to senior citizens about a 'Warm hearts, warm blankets' campaign. You'll soon find volunteers who can visit the wards, document the number of elderly patients left cold, and make sure they all have warm blankets. The local knitting or sewing group would probably be delighted to make and donate bedcovers.

7. Create the pathways

A notable feature of Tiritiri Matangi Island is the miles of tracks volunteers have built so visitors can enjoy the different aspects of the island and its wildlife. In work on compassion in healthcare, we too need pathways to show us the way.

Les Todres and colleagues at the University of Bornemouth offer a value framework for guiding research and practice in the humanization of healthcare [19].

Each of the eight dimensions in the framework is seen as a continuum, stretching from a term that characterizes humanization in a positive sense through to a term that characterizes the barrier to such a possibility.

Forms of humanization	Forms of dehumanization
Insiderness	Objectification
Agency	Passivity
Uniqueness	Homogenization
Togetherness	Isolation
Sense-making	Loss of meaning
Personal journey	Loss of personal journey
Sense of place	Dislocation
Embodiment	Reductionist body

The power of these dimensions is seen when we consider the typical hospital ward round, with the doctors and other health professionals clustered around a patient's bed.

Very often the professionals speak across the bed as if the patient didn't exist – passivity and isolation. The patient is referred to by the name of the disease – objectification, loss of personal journey.

Test results and treatments are discussed – homogenization and reductionist body, in language the patient cannot understand – loss of meaning, dislocation.

The authors of this framework are not suggesting a dualism – that each dimension of care is either humanized or not – but instead that we judge where on the spectrum each instance of caring lies.

Imagine a consultation where a deeply empathetic nurse or physician built a caring partnership with the patient and family, allowing the patient to set the agenda, learning much about the meaning and context of the illness in the patient's life, and developing an holistic plan of treatment and support recognizing the unique personal circumstances.

Todres's dimensions serve as a useful checklist when too often our improvement efforts focus only on process design, clinical performance and safety, without considering how does the interaction feel to the patient?

8. Conduct scientific studies of behavior to inform your work

On Tiritiri Matangi Island there is an extensive scientific research program, developing the knowledge about the best ways to restore the natural ecosystem and conserve endangered species. Likewise, our efforts to re-humanize healthcare and to restore a healing environment need to be informed by field research in the patient care environment.

Paul Bate and Glen Robert are renowned for their application of Experience Based Design (EBD) to healthcare improvement [20].

> "We suggest that designing services, environments, interactions and processes for the human experience – literally targeting experience – poses a formidable, but highly worthwhile, challenge for healthcare improvement professionals.

> "This is not just about being more patient-centered or promoting greater patient participation. It goes much further than this, placing the experience goals of patients and users at the center of the design process and on the same footing as process and clinical goals."

When patients tell stories about their interaction with healthcare services, intensely personal points on the journey are revealed that represent key moments that stand out as crucial to their experience. Bate and Robert call these touch points – those times when a patient recalls being touched emotionally or cognitively, forming deep and lasting memories.

Identifying touch points is central to the process of Experience Based Design. Only the patient holds this knowledge but when health professionals work with patients as co-designers of an improved service, exploring the meaning of these touch points yields unique and precious insights that can help transform care.

> "Stories and storytelling are the basis of experience design. As the repository of experience, they contain almost everything that is required for a deep appreciative understanding of the strengths and weaknesses of a present service and of what needs to be redesigned for the future."

Belinda Dewar and colleagues at the Leadership in Compassionate Care Programme in Edinburgh used emotional touch points and appreciative inquiry to draw out patient experiences [21].

Because people often lack a rich emotional vocabulary, Dewar used pre-printed cards showing a range of emotional words, both positive and negative, to prompt patients to identify how the experience felt to them. The cards had words like numb, powerless, bewildered, happy, curious, hopeful, unsure, enjoyment, satisfied, reluctant, at ease, and encouraged.

Asking patients to identify the emotions connected with their experience often challenged the pre-conceived ideas of health workers about patients' desires and preferences. One patient chose cards with the words: surprised, enjoyment, at ease, when she told this story:

"One of the staff on the ward came up to me the other day and asked if I wanted to move into a side room so that I could get more sleep at night and feel more rested during the day. I was surprised to be offered this.

"One of the ladies opposite me has dementia and she calls out at night a lot and goes into other people's lockers and takes things. I don't mind though. I like to be in her company. I have a good friend at home who has dementia and I enjoy spending time with her. It does not bother me. I don't want to go to the side room. I feel at ease with Janet."

The woman's response challenged staff's assumptions about what it was like to be with a person who behaved in different ways, and prompted staff to ensure that they always checked with patients when making any decisions about moving patients.

In the process of appreciative inquiry, three main action-reflection cycles emerged in identifying the compassionate care processes that are important for staff, patients and families [22]:

1.   Knowing who I am and what matters to me

2.   Understanding how I feel

3.   Working with me to shape the ways things are done

When staff were asked to reflect on the outcomes of the program they talked about caring for and about each other; being conscious about giving positive feedback; valuing, legitimizing, and articulating compassionate caring acts; feeling confident to speak out and ask questions about the way we do things around here; and being curious and taking another look at what we do.

9. Learn from others

Tiritiri Matangi Island is just one of many conservation sites linked across the world. These pioneering efforts are linked together by knowledge sharing and exchange of staff and resources. We can do the same in healthcare.

The mission of the Schwartz Center for Compassionate Healthcare in Boston is to promote compassionate healthcare so patients and caregivers relate in a way that provides hope to the patient, support to the caregiver and sustenance to the healing process [23].

The Center trains health professionals in spiritual caregiving skills; makes grants to health providers to sponsor Compassion Rounds; has a Speaker Series; and Compassionate Caregiving awards.

Schwartz Center Rounds are now established in more than 240 health care facilities. Rather like a hospital Grand Round, a clinical team presents a patient case history to an interdisciplinary audience. However, rather than the clinical and technical details of care, the focus is on the human dimensions of medicine, the social and emotional issues that arise in caring for patients.

A retrospective evaluation of the Rounds showed participants were more likely to attend psychosocial and emotional aspects of care and enhanced their beliefs about the importance of empathy [24]. Respondents reported better teamwork, including heightened appreciation of the roles and contributions of colleagues. There were significant decreases in stress and improvements in the ability to cope with the psychosocial demands of care.

The Point of Care programme [25] at the King's Fund in London aims, to help health care staff in hospitals deliver the quality of care they would want for themselves and their own families.

The group works with patients and their families, staff and hospital boards to research, test and share new approaches to improving patients' experience.

The website (kingsfund.org.uk/current_projects/point_of_care/) offers access to workshops, reports and other resources for learning and collaboration. They also promote Experience Based Design and Schwartz Center Rounds in the UK.

The bigger picture

Stepping aside from our analogy of the conservation island, we have to answer two questions from our skeptical healthcare leaders:

'How can we afford the time and resources needed to strengthen compassion and caring when we have already overspent our budget?'

'And how will we know we made any difference? Can you even measure compassion?'

I'll address these two questions in turn.

How can we afford the investment in time and resources?

By now I'm hoping that you are convinced strengthening compassion and caring generates benefits for your bottom line:

- Better clinical outcomes, fewer complications, shorter patient stays

- Greater patient satisfaction, more trust, better adherence to treatment

- Fewer patients suing you, less damages to pay out

- Enhanced reputation, more business, and ability to attract the best health professionals

- Happier workers, less sickness and absenteeism, reduced staff turnover

It's estimated the true cost of replacing one experienced staff nurse is between $20,000 and $40,000 when you take into account advertising and recruitment costs, temporary staffing, agency fees, administrative costs, orientation and training.

If you are losing fifteen or twenty percent of your staff each year – not unusual in today's stressed healthcare system – the cost to your organization may run into millions of dollars per year.

Investing in the health, wellbeing and happiness of workers by creating the conditions where they reconnect to the heart of their practice – is an investment with a high and immediate rate of return.

And compassionate care may actually be cheaper, particularly end-of-life care.

Palliative Care

Too often I see patients having an undignified and tortured death in an acute hospital setting, while doctors continue the fight to preserve life long after there is any hope of survival.

Even when the patient, family and doctor are all agreed that the patient is in a terminal phase of illness and that the case is hopeless, I see patients treated to death with drugs, needles, infusions, blood tests, and all the other paraphernalia of modern technical care.

The feeling I get is that doctors can't bear to do nothing; that somehow giving up all the rituals of treatment is admitting a terrible defeat.

This is the result of a dehumanized system where health workers don't have the necessary wellbeing, attitudes and skills to provide love, compassion, kindness and comfort to a dying patient.

Very often it's the patient and family who demand of the doctor, 'Do everything possible!' even when the patient has no chance of surviving.

Why does this happen? It's because neither the doctor nor the family have the necessary support to guide the difficult conversation about death and dying. So in their shared vulnerability and fear, they egg each other on in distressing parodies of care.

This cycle of fear and insecurity is responsible for an enormous burden of unproductive healthcare expenditure. Billions of dollars are spent on inhumane end-of-life hospital care when a much better way exists. This is one area where compassionate caring can save enormous sums of money.

Physicians and nurses who are experts in palliative care have radically different kinds of conversations with dying patients and their families. Instead of a relentless focus on trying yet another futile treatment to stave off the inevitable – often at the cost of severe side effects – these compassionate and humane practitioners are able to explore the patient's own goals at end of life.

How can a patient making the most of the precious few weeks or months, to connect with family and friends, reflect on a life, and focus on what is most important?

When patient and families are given this support, they clarify personal goals and make very different choices about care. Very often they reject yet another round of futile chemotherapy, forgo the surgery or intensive care, and choose instead to spend their time at home, living life to the fullest.

A research study across eight hospitals in the USA compared costs of care for patients who had access to palliative care consultations, with those who had 'usual care' [26].

Those palliative care patients discharged alive had an adjusted net savings of $1696 in direct costs per hospital admission, and those who died during the admission had an adjusted net savings of $4908 in direct costs.

There were significant reductions in pharmacy, laboratory and intensive care costs compared with usual care patients.

This cheaper care is also better care. Palliative care is shown to improve physical and psychological symptom management for the patient, enhance caregiver wellbeing, and improve family satisfaction.

More recently a randomized controlled trial showed that patients receiving early palliative care for metastatic lung cancer actually survived longer than patients given aggressive cancer treatment [27].

Palliative care patients had a better quality of life, a much lower incidence of depression (16% versus 38%) and lived on average 11.6 months compared with 8.9 months.

More care is not better care. In today's environment of rapidly escalating healthcare costs, the question is not, 'How can we afford compassionate care?' Rather the question is, 'How can we afford NOT to re-humanize our healthcare system?'

How will we know we have made a difference?

Many times people have asked me, 'How can you measure compassion?' Or else, 'If you can't measure it, how will you know you have made a difference?'

Others have argued that attempting to measure something as elusive as compassion will debase or destroy the very quality we are trying to encourage.

I take a pragmatic view. For frightened and vulnerable patients meeting a physician or nurse for the first time it's blindingly obvious to them, within a minute or two of the encounter, whether their caregiver truly cares. The ultimate test must be the subjective quality of the patient's experience.

In our work to re-humanize healthcare we are seeking four major shifts:

Reductionist focus on pathology	➤ Focus on whole person
Detached care	➤ Empathetic, compassionate care
Focus on sickness, defects and problems	➤ Focus on wellbeing, strengths and resilience
Health professional directing care	➤ Health professional serving the patient's goals

These four dimensions comprise what might be called the 'Technical-Human Continuum'.

Although it's possible for a physician or surgeon immersed in technical medicine to also be a humanistic practitioner who sees the whole person, by and large the practitioner's behavior on these four dimensions are correlated.

The deeply humane physician who humbly serves the goals of his or her patient is unlikely to see the pathology as isolated from the patient's lifestyle, relationships, thoughts and emotions.

And the detached clinician who has mastered the latest hi-tech treatment is unlikely to focus on the wellbeing, strengths and resilience of his patient.

So although the social scientists may throw their arms in the air, protesting about the invalidity of measuring one value to represent a multidimensional construct, I think in real life patients will have little difficulty with this measure:

How do you rate your care by making a mark somewhere on this line?

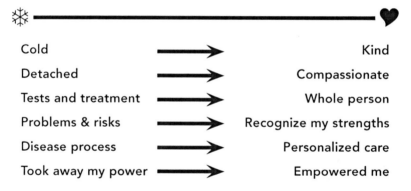

So, here's our challenge:

Will we aspire to compassionate caring that improves the quality of our patients' lives, achieves higher satisfaction, fewer complications, less cost, and allows our patients to live longer? As health professionals do we want to find again the joy and satisfaction in our work?

Or do we continue this headlong rush towards ever more expensive, inhumane, and technological treatment – deluding ourselves that this is caring?

Chapter 11

COMPASSIONATE LEADERSHIP

Leadership in healthcare can be a difficult and dangerous business.

A close friend grew up as the son of medical missionaries. His childhood influences show up in his medical practice, offering low-cost care to large numbers of patients. He undercuts the local private surgeons, charging for his procedures about one tenth of their rates.

The reward for his compassionate caring and public service is persecution by the greedy surgeons, who turn patients against him, question his competence, and sponsor vexatious complaints about him to the medical authorities.

Business and medicine are poor bedfellows. When doctors seek to maximize their income, rather than do what is best for their patient, a serious conflict of interest arises.

Much of the excessive and harmful activity in healthcare is driven by the profit motive, linked to fee-for-service payment schedules.

So if you stand up for caring, compassion and the humble service of patients and communities, you are a threat to established and powerful interests.

Even within public hospitals and clinics, where personal profit motives are largely absent, compassionate caring may draw fire.

You may be criticized for being weak, soft, for wasting time and letting patients manipulate you. It's sad to see health professionals become disillusioned and cynical but that's the reality in many workplaces.

Our language shapes our assumptions and beliefs

One of my medical colleagues is a pioneer in Emergency Medicine. He's worked a lifetime in many ER's in the USA. He says that in every hospital he worked in, the senior ER nurses were battle-hardened and cynical. In Britain the ER is often called the 'Casualty Department'. It's a fitting title for a place that on a Saturday evening more resembles a war zone than a place of healing.

In fact, the corporate culture that has pervaded so many health providers is full of military and machine language. It's contaminating the world of healthcare and is reflected in our battle cries like 'winning the war on cancer!' or 'winning the war on drugs!'

Stop, for a moment, to reflect on the language we unconsciously use each day in healthcare:

We talk about workforce and manpower

We manage workload and outputs

We are led by chief executive officers

We implement strategies and execute plans

We use techniques and toolkits

We triage patients in the casualty department

And we shoot home the message by using bullet points on PowerPoint slides!

The language we use powerfully shapes our thoughts and actions. And what we focus on comes into being, which is why Mother Teresa said she would never demonstrate against war but the moment there was a rally for peace she would be there.

If we wish to create compassionate places of healing, we need to moderate our language and shift away from our unconscious assumptions of mechanistic control and authority.

These expressions have infiltrated healthcare from the competitive world of big business. Are these the values we want in healthcare? What different kind of language could our leaders use to signal a shift?

These are the words I want to hear from my leaders because they will resonate with my heart and remind me why I came into healthcare:

- Compassion
- Caring
- Understanding and loving kindness
- Collaboration
- Partnership
- Community and shared belonging
- Meaning, purpose and spirit

When we declare war, we create opposition. When we command others, we create resistance. If instead we bring mindful attention to our spirit and our words, we find a gentler way.

There is a natural power for healing. The wise leader or physician or nurse knows how much can be achieved by so little, when there is alignment of thoughts, intentions, words and actions. Gandhi said, 'We must be the change we want to see'.

But Ghandi also advocated civil disobedience. There is a fine balance. I think there is some room for compassionate disobedience!

The hero leader

It's taken me a long time to begin to understand this gentler concept of leadership. My bookshelves are filled with books on management and leadership and many of them corrupted my thoughts and beliefs about the best way to lead change.

Many writers have contrasted the role of managers and leaders.

Managers take a complicated project and specify the steps to achieve the project outcomes. They use authority to direct resources to complete tasks and hold people accountable for performance on tasks – including sticking to the budget.

Leaders, on the other hand, make sure we are doing the right project in the first place. Their broad view of future possibilities gives us a sense of shared direction and purpose. Where managers command, leaders persuade.

Actually, the distinction between managers and leaders is unhelpful because all good managers lead, and all good leaders manage. It's much more helpful to consider management and leadership as roles, rather than to stereotype individuals.

In a hierarchical view of organizations, the leaders are perceived to be the people at the top, the smart ones with the great ideas. At least in the Western world, we are very stuck on the hero model of leadership.

After the 1990-1 Gulf war, General Norman "Stormin" Schwarzkopf was feted as a hero by business leaders who paid up to $1,000 for the privilege of hearing him speak about leadership, and $10,000 to sit at his dinner table.

If you look at the business section in any bookshop, you'll find numerous books on leadership extolling the virtues of heroic individuals like Jack Welsh, the CEO of General Electric, and Rudy Giuliani the Mayor of New York City at the time of the 9-11 terrorist attacks on the World Trade Center.

Even in literature about leadership in the public and political domain, you'll find accounts of heroic individuals like civil rights leader Martin Luther King. His speech, 'I have a dream' is held up as one of the most inspirational speeches of all time.

For many years I had a notion of leadership that encompassed visionary ideas, powerful rhetoric, and the ability to persuade others.

The dangers of persuasion

In the late 1990's I was invited to address the national forum of Chief Medical Officers in New Zealand, at a time when the public health service was under threat because the government believed healthcare would be more efficient if hospital leadership was corporatized.

Clinical leaders were disenfranchised and the medical profession had fallen into a state of helplessness and blaming. The government reforms had placed captains of industry in the public health service, displacing the medical directors and chief nurses who previously led the hospitals.

In response, I had created a national association of clinical leaders in an attempt to show that health professionals could still be proactive in the leadership of health service improvements.

When I spoke at the Chief Medical Officers' forum, two of the attendees congratulated me on my energy and passion – it was something desperately needed in the health system, they said.

Another attendee, a cardiologist, remarked drily that he preferred to call my attitude "evangelical enthusiasm". Little did I know it at the time, but this character was to become a powerful adversary.

Two years later, I quit my job at a big teaching hospital to take up a leadership role in the development of a small community hospital, serving an underprivileged community. The creation of this hospital was bitterly opposed by the Clinical Director of Medicine – none other than the cardiologist who had disparaged my passion and energy.

He believed splitting services across two sites would be very damaging. He worked in a bigger hospital in the richest and healthiest community in New Zealand, the opposite side of the city from the disadvantaged community where I lived.

I believed our community was best served by having a local hospital, and knew that many residents could not even afford the cost of the ambulance trip across town. As a cardiologist, his major concern was the efficient provision of specialist services within the hospital.

To my eyes, the Clinical Director of medicine was arrogant, patronizing, and paternalistic; he apparently had little insight into the impact of social disadvantage and cultural differences on health outcomes.

Some of his patient loved him - those patients who wanted an old school, authoritarian doctor, buttoned up in a white coat. The patients who wanted to make their own healthcare decisions told me they found him overbearing and difficult.

He argued that the best care for an eighty-year-old patient with multiple pathologies was to divide care among the cardiologist, respiratory physician, renal specialist, endocrinologist, rheumatologist, and psychiatrist. He quoted research showing that specialists provided a better standard of care than generalists.

In this reductionist and fragmented model of care, I wondered where was the doctor who saw the whole person?

For several years I'd worked as Intern Supervisor looking after the wellbeing of our most junior doctors at the smaller hospital. I saw the new hospital as an opportunity to redesign the model of teamwork, so interns could be part of an inter-disciplinary team focused on the patients needs. I was deeply dismayed therefore when the Clinical Director of Medicine imposed an outdated model.

This traditional model of the 'medical team' left inexperienced doctors caring for the sickest patients, often without any practical supervision. Their workloads in the evenings, nights and weekends were inhuman. As Clinical Leader of the hospital, I had investigated numerous poor patient outcomes and knew the threat to patient safety posed by such outdated models.

Moreover, I was a member of the national committee advising the New Zealand Government on healthcare quality and safety and also the NZ representative on a World Health Organization International Steering Committee on Patient Safety Solutions. I thought I knew what I was talking about.

Fortunately, the chief executive of the health board at that time knew that a different kind of approach was needed to meet the needs of the poor community we served. The new smaller hospital was given a degree of autonomy and for many years I worked with an inspirational general manager and a wonderful director of nursing. We worked arduously to create a more humane, safe and compassionate workplace.

I lobbied hard for an integrated medical model, where a core of dedicated physicians could build the relationships with other departments on the site of our little hospital. My nemesis insisted that physicians from the Department of Medicine could only staff our hospital in a strict, six-monthly rotation from the big hospital.

Over the years we won supporters to our cause. One by one, we persuaded individual physicians that our hospital was a great place to work; that caring for the whole patient was more satisfying than merely treating pathology; that humbly serving our diverse community was a satisfying challenge.

The point of this tale is to illustrate the hazards of an oppositional style of leadership.

I thought my job as a leader was to persuade people to change. I was righteous in my defense of the local hospital and our community and was critical of the attitudes and practices of many of my fellow doctors.

In the process I demonized the role of my adversary.

In truth, he was a kind, caring and deeply committed doctor who selflessly worked at the big hospital all hours of the day and night. When a junior doctor called for help, he would attend unhesitatingly. The nurses on the coronary care unit adored him. For his sixtieth birthday, they created a humorous calendar with photos of the nurses dressed up in provocative poses.

Even though he opposed the development of our new hospital, he insisted his physicians take part in the medical staff roster. He rostered himself on-call for the first month of our brand-new coronary care unit and oversaw the opening of the new medical wards.

When a new chief executive was appointed at the health board, disaster struck. The inspirational leadership team at the smaller hospital was torn apart in a management restructure. I lost my role as clinical leader. Most of the managers and leaders with the biggest hearts, who cared the most about the local community, lost their jobs. The smaller hospital became a satellite to the big hospital across the other side of the city.

I wrote to the new chief executive expressing serious concerns about patient safety and requested a meeting. I had enjoyed a close relationship with the previous chief executive and Board members. The new chief executive refused to see me, saying I should present my concerns to my general manager.

I responded by explaining that the most serious cause of patient safety problems was the lack of collaboration among the different medical services, headed by different general managers. Only he as chief executive could address this over-arching organizational problem. I also pointed out I was a national authority on patient safety.

He again refused to meet with me. Soon after, he announced the management restructure. I never again had contact with the Executive Team or the Board. I was persona non grata, the Latin phrase which translates "an unwelcome person".

Leadership without persuasion

Thankfully, many positive changes endured after the leaders were banished. In fact, this might be the ultimate test of leadership: do others still uphold the gains when you are long gone?

When people walk into our community hospital they still sense a positive atmosphere. People greet them with a smile and friendly offer of help. Most health workers enjoy their jobs and patient complaints are rare.

The most profound change occurred in the maternity service. Patient care was threatened by a breakdown in the professional relationship between midwives and doctors, characterized by mutual blaming, recrimination and a lack of teamwork. We witnessed a string of bad outcomes, morale collapsed, several practitioners faced professional investigation, and staffing levels reached critical levels.

Using the skills of a very gifted facilitator, we explored the conflicting professional beliefs and set up a monthly dialogue group. Over a period of two years, trust was rebuilt, teamwork enhanced and working relationships were transformed.

The hospital's cesarean section rate fell by thirty percent, the number of neonates with poor birth condition dramatically reduced, staffing levels were restored, and the rate of patient complaints fell dramatically [1].

When I eventually left the hospital, we had a farewell dinner in the maternity department. Among the twenty-five people who attended were many of the leaders and participants of those dramatic events ten years before, who still worked at the hospital.

What's interesting about the work in the maternity department is that none of the leaders made any attempt to persuade others about the 'right' answers.

Our role as leaders was to act as host and facilitators of the process of change, while solutions naturally emerged from the dialogue and the shared desire of all to care better for mothers and babies.

On the other hand, many of the gains we made in other areas, through advocacy and persuasion, were eroded after the leaders left.

What this experience suggests, is that heroic models of leadership may not be the best way to create sustainable change within complex systems like healthcare. In chapter 13, *Hearts in Healthcare*, I further explore the idea of the leader as 'host' rather than 'hero'.

If you are reading this book, you are probably passionate about trying to strengthen caring and compassion in healthcare. Perhaps you have had an experience of being a patient or seeing a loved one suffer in an uncaring institution? Maybe you are just someone who is unusually sensitive and empathetic, who feels the suffering of patients and is deeply concerned about the wellbeing of your fellow health professionals?

Your passion and concern are both an asset and a liability. Your passion will keep you going, year-after-year, within institutions whose leaders value productivity, achieving targets, and keeping within budget, more than love for patients. But the strength of your feelings may precipitate conflict, isolation and even marginalization, unless you can find supportive networks of like-minded individuals.

The problem of problem-solving

In addition to the unhelpful Western models of leadership, steeped in visionary and heroic roles, we're also bedeviled with improvement strategies that focus relentlessly on problem solving.

This problem-focused approach to healthcare improvement is woven into the fabric of everyday work because our whole patient care strategy is based on identifying pathologies (problems) and risks.

We have a sickness system rather than a health system because instead of focusing on the strengths, resilience and adaptability of our patients we look for defects and risks. This approach is reflected in our problem-based medical records and problem-based learning.

If you put any groups of health professionals in a room and ask them how we can improve patient flow through the emergency department they'll come up with a list of problems – most caused by someone else! It's rare for anyone to say, 'On this day the system worked exceptionally well. I wonder if we can identify the factors that created success on that day?'

So a very helpful leadership strategy is to make people aware of their unconscious thinking styles.

The famous pioneer of lateral thinking, Edward de Bono, wrote about thinking styles in his immensely helpful book, *Six Thinking Hats* [2].

Where traditional Western thinking assigned attributes like optimism, pessimism and creativity to individual personalities – de Bono proposed that workgroups could deliberately consider every angle, by mentally donning different colored hats.

So 'yellow hat' thinking is focusing on the benefits and advantages of a proposed change. And 'green hat' thinking is a process of creativity and brainstorming.

When de Bono described 'black-hat thinking' – a critical and pessimistic thinking style, focusing on problems and risks – it was physicians he was imagining!

Of course, black-hat thinking is enormously valuable for physicians and engineers – we want our patients to be safe and bridges to be strong – but it's not the only thinking style that exists. De Bono argued that it needs to be balanced with more positive and creative thinking styles.

It amuses me now to understand how completely unconscious I was of my black-hat thinking style, and the problems it caused in the early days of my marriage.

My wife suggested remodeling the kitchen at home. I thought she had some great ideas but my immediate and unconscious response was to highlight all the problems with her proposal!

We ended up arguing and she fled in tears, convinced I wanted to undermine her ideas.

I was bewildered by her reaction because I was just figuring out how to make her idea work by identifying the problems that would need solving. (I'm an engineer AND a doctor, so you can guess how 'black-hat' I was).

It took me a long time to adopt a 'yellow-hat' and respond more positively to her smart suggestions, while putting forward constructive ideas about solving some of the problems. I'd have to say that shifting my attitude is still a work in progress, so deeply ingrained are the habits of thought.

Learning about thinking hats was a vivid illustration for me about how unconsciously our assumptions, habits, frameworks and thinking styles shape our responses to situations.

Appreciative Inquiry

In healthcare improvement efforts, the most powerful way to overcome the difficulties of critical thinking is a wonderful process called Appreciative Inquiry.

You'll recall from chapter 10 that Belinda Dewar and her colleagues at the Leadership in Compassionate Care Programme in Edinburgh are keen advocates of this approach [3].

It's used successfully in many organizations around the world but has hardly touched healthcare.

The major pioneers in Appreciative Inquiry are a visionary team of health professionals at the University of Virginia Health System. In 2011 they published the first book on the application of AI to healthcare improvement, *Appreciative Inquiry in Healthcare. Positive Questions to Bring Out the Best* [4].

I have to admit, as an engineer turned physician, I was deeply skeptical on first learning about Appreciative Inquiry. How can a process of deliberately ignoring problems yield anything useful in healthcare?

The first answer is that it works. Magically. The authors illustrate their text with many deeply moving stories but it's their success in building collaboration among widely diverse participants that is striking. The process works in any setting.

From the cardiovascular operating room team, interventional radiology, the medical school admissions committee, the rehabilitation hospital, the school of nursing, right through to the department of neurology. Other departments clamor to be the next in line, to join in to this energizing and exciting process.

The second answer is deeper. Those who work in healthcare tend to see the world as a very concrete reality. We invest much effort in objectivity, measurement and precision of problem definition. We tend to externalize problems and figure out solutions. Yet it turns out that much of our reality is of our own making.

Just as atoms materialize into particles the moment we turn on a particle detector, and behave like waves when we look for interference patterns, the lens we choose defines the world we see. When we focus on problems and risks, we lose creativity and imagination. People feel threatened, defend their own practice and resort to blaming others for defects in care.

Creativity and imagination start to bloom. People begin to dream of a better future and work together to create it. That is the art of appreciative inquiry

But when we ask people to share stories of their peak experiences – when teamwork and care worked exceptionally well, when work assumed deep meaning and purpose, when people felt joyful and energized – then a different kind of energy arises. Creativity and imagination start to bloom. People begin to dream of a better future and work together to create it. That is the art of appreciative inquiry.

You'll notice that this idea is strongly supported by the findings of positive psychology and Fredrickson's broaden-and-build theory of positive emotions: They open our hearts and minds thus making us more receptive, more creative and then allow us to discover and build new skills, new ties, new knowledge, and new ways of being [5].

The primary authors of Appreciative Inquiry are not management consultants but senior clinicians deeply involved in day-to-day patient care and bed-side teaching at a major academic medical center.

Their hands-on experience of using AI in real clinical and academic settings gives them great credibility.

More than that, they write from their hearts and inspire us with a vision of a workplace where caring, compassion and excellence in patient care are the things that flourish.

Appreciative Inquiry includes comprehensive strategies for organizational change in a 4-D cycle:

1. **Discovery:** What gives life? Appreciating
2. **Dreams:** What could be? Imagining
3. **Design:** What should be? Innovating
4. **Destiny:** What will we do? Delivering

The reasons that AI works so powerfully are multiple. People work at their best when they are optimistic, energized and focused on their strengths. Secondly, AI creates collaboration by engaging diverse participants in a way that avoids blaming and defensiveness. Thirdly, when questions like this are used in AI, they uncover deep meaning in work for both individuals and the broader organization. Finally, AI encourages people to share stories that engage the heart, not just the head.

Such approaches will avoid all the mistakes I made in the early days of my leadership efforts, which created opposition and resistance.

So instead of persuading people to change, you can offer open invitations to engage in different kinds of conversations. Whoever turns up will be the perfect people to support your cause! In my own hospital I began Compassion Rounds, inspired by the work of the Schwartz Center for Compassionate Care [6].

Similar to a hospital Grand Round, the compassion round begins with a case presentation and is intended for a multidisciplinary audience. In contrast to most Grand Rounds, which focus on the clinical and technical aspects of patient care, the Compassion Round explores the human dimension of care.

Schwartz Center Rounds have been adopted in many hundreds of hospitals and research shows they have many benefits in enhancing patient-centered communication, teamwork, and provider support [7].

Unlike the formal Schwartz Center Rounds, which rely on organizational commitment and a medical team roster for case presentations, we simply announced a monthly lunchtime meeting and provided a free lunch. Participants were invited to share stories and many moving dialogues occurred. We'd often have forty or fifty people attending.

As the word spread, more and more doctors started attending. One of the striking features was the cross-divisional attendance.

No other meeting in the hospital drew people together from medicine, maternity, psychiatry, pediatrics, surgery, and community services. Gatherings like this are a good way to identify other champions for compassionate care. You are not alone!

Nothing to lose

When you are inspired to become a champion for compassionate care and step up to lead positive change, here are two more thoughts about leadership.

The first is letting go.

I once had the privilege of attending a long weekend leadership retreat of twelve people, coached by the wonderful Margaret Wheatley. She's a deeply spiritual person who is a thought leader in community leadership and whole-system change, and a best-selling author [8].

On the second day, Wheatley split us into four groups of three and asked us to share one question with each other: "When were you most effective in your leadership? How did that come about?"

You'll notice she was using the power of appreciative inquiry!

I shared a story about suddenly finding myself the Acting Chair of a national committee in crisis. The Chair had resigned and we were faced with giving an ultimatum to the Minister of Health, or all resigning.

Another companion told an inspiring story about stepping up to save an indigenous TV channel when the newly appointed chief executive was found to have made a fraudulent application. When we joined back in the circle of twelve, we shared all of our stories. Every single tale had a common theme: in the crisis situations we individually faced, we all felt we had nothing to lose.

Having nothing to lose made us courageous in our leadership. It gave us unsuspected power. Clarity of position, shared commitment, and swift and decisive action led us all to success in our various ventures.

Our national committee won political support, a huge boost in funding, and gained wider powers through a revised Terms of Reference signed off by Cabinet.

Having nothing to lose made us courageous in our leadership. It gave us unsuspected power

The indigenous TV channel went on to become a highly successful public broadcast channel, admired for its diverse content and unique perspectives on current affairs.

As health professionals we invest so much in our professional training, our jobs, our roles and our status.

When I resigned my staff position as an anesthesiologist at the big teaching hospital in 2000, my colleagues were frankly disbelieving. Why would I want to give up my specialist skills to do an ordinary bread-and-butter job in a small hospital?

Sometimes we cling on to ideas. For more than a decade I strongly believed that the organizations I set up to improve healthcare should be non-profit, charitable bodies – particularly for the work on compassion in healthcare. I had this notion that compassion costs nothing and I wanted to separate it from the dirty world of profit.

That idea held me back for years. When I began to consider other options, many new opportunities arose.

The wonderful thing about letting go of ideas, status, identity or position is the way the Universe responds with such generosity.

Without fail, when I have finally let go of some cherished position or belief, then in a very short time completely new, unseen, and greater opportunities magically appear.

When we cling so hard to positions and beliefs, we become seriously blinkered. Our range of vision is narrowed and we become constrained in our imagination and our actions.

For a long time it was unthinkable that I could abandon my highly specialized professional work in the major teaching hospital. After all, I had invested fourteen years of incredibly hard work to achieve that elevated position.

But the moment I stepped away from that role, a whole new world opened up.

Unseen connections

When you commit to doing good in the world, and have the courage to let go of your previous identity and status, it's as if a force-field of good intention spreads around you, encouraging others to join your cause. People just show up unexpectedly.

This second idea is called "synchronicity".

Time and again, I have noticed that exactly the right person turns up to help you, just when you need it. The connections appear as if by some divine process of coincidence – synchronicity in action.

An inspiring account of just such a journey of leadership is *Synchronicity. The Inner Path of Leadership* by Joseph Jaworski [9].

When I began plans to create HEARTS in HEALTHCARE and had ideas of a world-wide online network, I wrote to several web development companies in Auckland. I figured that the project would go better if my collaborators were close to home. Not one of the companies even replied to my query.

Time and again, I have noticed that exactly the right person turns up to help you, just when you need them

Having quit my full-time job, I had signed on with a locum agency to do short-term placements in anesthesiology in the smaller hospitals around New Zealand, wherever there are staff shortages.

My first placement was in Invercargill, in the deep south of the South Island, a cold and wind-swept place especially in the middle of winter. I had never been to that part of the country before. I found the coolness of the climate was contrasted with the warmth and genuineness of the people.

Still frustrated with the lack of a web designer, I did a Google search for experts in Drupal (the open-source software I wanted to use) and found a company called Bluff IT. Bluff is the southernmost town in New Zealand, famous for its oysters. I was amused that a company would call itself 'bluff it'. It suggested a lack of pretension.

I went for a visit and met the sole proprietor sitting in the kitchen of an historic old homestead, which he and his partner had restored to become Bed & Breakfast accommodation. Andrew McClure has been one of my wonderful discoveries.

Not only has he done a wonderful job project managing the complex software development but he also recommended other team members: In nearby Invercargill I found a wonderful graphic design company, Emotive Design. They share offices with a small company called Write Answers who are experts in writing, editing, media relations, and promotion.

All of these people are passionate about the HEARTS in HEALTHCARE work. They are honest, unpretentious, down-to-earth and have overheads that are a small fraction of the expensive companies in Auckland.

The happy chances have continued to multiply. A trip to give a keynote address at a conference in Sydney led to a lunchtime conversation, an introduction, and an invitation to visit the home of the person who became the first major investor in HEARTS in HEALTHCARE.

Commitment

The journey of leadership begins with commitment. In chapter 3 I told the tale of Justin Micalizzi, the young boy who died as a result of medical error. His mother Dale has yet to receive any explanation or apology for his death.

In the years that have passed, Micalizzi has become a powerful advocate for safe, compassionate, patient centered healthcare and resolution of issues around medical errors through full disclosure. Justin's Hope Project focuses on HOPE: Healthcare Openness, Professionalism and Excellence [10].

Micalizzi offers a leadership challenge in memory of her son, with a call to personal integrity:

> "The highest courage is to dare to be yourself in the face of adversity. Choosing right over wrong, ethics over convenience, and truth over popularity... these are the choices that measure your life. Travel the path of integrity without looking back, for there is never a wrong time to do the right thing."

Chapter 12

PERSONAL TURNING POINT

I hope by now that you're convinced that a re-humanized healthcare system, that emphasizes compassion and caring, is going to be good for everyone. I believe it's the only solution to a rapidly escalating crisis in healthcare.

Healthcare faces a moral crisis: many health professionals have lost meaning and purpose in their work, and there are high rates of disillusionment, depression and burnout. Moreover, the commercialization of healthcare, professional self-interest and greed are corrupting the humanistic values of patient care – altruism, compassion, caring, and the desire to be of service to the community.

And there is a practical crisis too: Healthcare is broke. There is no more money to satisfy the rapidly rising costs of healthcare, already amounting to 17% of GDP in the USA. To that is added a health workforce crisis. Many health providers are cutting back services because they cannot find the doctors, nurses and other health workers they need to sustain care.

The only person who can make this change is you. And when enough people like you choose this different path, then the whole system will change

So a renewed healthcare system that restores the joy and satisfaction of health workers, that achieves better outcomes at lower cost, that strengthens the desire to serve, and that empower patients to maintain their own health and wellbeing – that would be an attractive solution, right?

This revolution will not come about through government healthcare reform, legislative change, or reworking of payment systems.

The only person who can make this change is you. And when enough people like you choose this different path, then the whole system will change.

This chapter is about finding your personal turning point, beyond which your work and your life will begin to flourish. Here is the pathway to happiness, wellbeing and resilience – not only for yourself but for your patients too.

I'd like to tell you a story of how one of my colleagues found her turning point.

It's like I have a new job!

A troubled hospital where I worked for many years lurched from crisis to crisis. Stories of poor patient care filled the front page of the local newspaper, culminating in a Commission of Enquiry into the care of frail elderly patients. Morale was terrible, and staff turnover had reached dangerous levels.

Mary (I have changed her name) is a senior health worker at this troubled hospital. Like many of her colleagues Mary admitted to feeling stressed, tired, disenchanted with her work, and heading for burnout. A single encounter with a patient changed all that.

Some months earlier, Mary had attended a workshop in which I used video film of patients telling their stories of what it's like to experience healthcare. Within the mixed group of health professionals we had discussed compassion, caring and kindness. For Mary, the seeds of change had been sown but it took a particular patient encounter for the real learning to occur.

Mary was referred to assess a frail old woman with multiple medical problems and partial blindness. When she began the bedside consultation, she noticed the patient was distressed. She paused and asked if there was something that she could do to help.

The patient hesitatingly told her that she was extremely worried about some circumstance at home and urgently needed to use the phone.

'Did you ask the ward nurses?' queried Mary.

'Yes,' said the old woman. 'I asked every day to use the cordless phone but they keep telling me that's only for staff and I should use the patients' card phone down the corridor.'

Her lips quivered and she tipped her shoulder in a helpless gesture. 'I can't use that phone, you see. I'm almost blind.'

Mary told me the situation had suddenly triggered a memory of the workshop discussion about simple acts of kindness. In that instant, she decided to act.

Excusing herself, Mary hurried to the hospital shop and purchased a phone card. Returning to the ward, she asked the old woman, 'Who is it that you need to call? I'll give you a hand'.

Mary led her to the phone and helped her make the connection. The patient cried with gratitude and relief. This was the first time in two weeks that anyone in the hospital had listened to her concerns.

What's more, for the first time since admission, the old patient's heart condition started to improve and she began a process of healing and recovery.

Mary reflected on this event during the day and talked about it at home. She came to realize that this simple act of kindness was the single most satisfying thing she had done at work for a long time. Lately she had been feeling tired and dispirited.

By the next morning, Mary had redefined her professional role: kindness first, expertise second. She promised to herself that she would look for an opportunity each day to perform an unexpected act of kindness.

As she told me this story, her eyes shone and her face became animated. 'It's like I have a new job,' she said.

I have told Mary's story countless times and it always stirs emotions in an audience of health professionals. Some shed tears.

So many of us are trying to find a place for our heart in an uncaring healthcare system. Mary's story gives us hope.

Mary still worked in the same hospital, in the same role. The job hadn't changed at all, but she had. She had learned the extraordinary power of performing simple acts of kindness for the patients in her care.

Choosing where we direct our attention

Even ten years ago, psychologists would have struggled to understand such a transformation. But if you have read all the earlier chapters, you'll now begin to understand how the rapidly expanding field of Positive Psychology is generating important new insights into happiness and wellbeing.

The key new understanding is we can reshape our minds by directing attention. Where our thoughts and intentions dwell has a major influence on feelings, perceptions and beliefs about the world.

Once Mary made a deliberate decision to seek out opportunities for small acts of kindness, it required a shift in her attention.

Previously, her mind was occupied with clinical tasks, alternating with an internal dialogue about the dissatisfactions in her life. She had angry thoughts about the frustrations of her job, the excessive demands, the difficult people she had to work with, and her feelings of tiredness and depression.

Now she was reprogrammed. The conscious effort to be more sensitive to the needs of her patients meant she began to notice more. And when she performed the little acts of kindness, her mind was suddenly flooded with positive thoughts and emotions.

It's a reprogramming that MIT Economist Dan Ariely explains in his 2008 book, *Predictably Irrational* [1]. Ariely was looking at why markets so frequently failed to follow the rules of supply and demand that economists had so sensibly laid out for them. Traditional economists had worked under a fallacy – they'd assumed that faced with a series of choices people would evaluate them rationally and select the one that represented best value.

When Ariely tested that theory he found that not only did people make decisions based more on emotion than logic, but that they also tended to make those same irrational decisions over and over again – what Ariely described as "lining up behind themselves".

Ariely's book explains how much our behavior is shaped by emotional responses and rewards, in self-reinforcing patterns, rather than rational decision-making.

The health worker who displays detached, impersonal care is more likely to elicit 'difficult' behavior from patients, which merely reinforces the need to remain detached. However, the empathetic, sensitive, kind health worker experiences a very different emotional response to his or her actions, reinforcing the positive behavior.

Having once made a decision to change her own behaviour, each time Mary was confronted with the same set of circumstances, she was likely to make the same choice.

When she tuned in her kindness radar, a very surprising thing happened. She noticed that many other people did kind things for her, holding a door open, finding the charts, introducing her to the patient, and empathizing with her. When she was so self-absorbed in both her tasks and her feelings of grumpiness she had never really noticed these kind acts before. Now her work environment began to feel like a much friendlier place.

Becoming the best version of ourselves

Over the years, hearing similar stories from many different health professionals, I began to wonder about the idea of a personal epiphany akin to the 'tipping point' Malcolm Gladwell popularized in his best-selling book of the same name. He described the conditions that result in a sudden new fashion sweeping the world, or mass uptake of a new idea or product [2].

What strikes me is the recurring theme of the stories: the triggering events are very small, they always involve a deep sense of connection with a patient, the effects are out of all proportion to the deed done, and the change once begun is irreversible – the health professional is never the same again.

The magical moment seems to trigger a fundamental shift, a new process of learning and change when health professionals suddenly find themselves on an upward spiral of flourishing.

These changes are also visible to others, especially patients. Some new aspect in the health professionals' attitude causes patients to respond differently. The result is an increased sense of connection, a greater joy and satisfaction in daily practice, and a reinforcement of the process of change.

Some new aspect in the health professionals' attitude causes patients to respond differently

Health professionals derive job satisfaction and interest from many sources, including the mastery of a complex art, gained through hard years of training and experience. There's no denying the satisfaction of a difficult task carried out with great skill, often in difficult circumstances. But in the end, technical skills are often not enough to keep us happy in our practice.

Sometimes the greatest healing can arise from doing nothing, simply bearing witness to suffering. But doing nothing is against our nature.

Our healthcare culture is one of doing: questioning, examining, testing, diagnosing, treating and caring. With the unrelenting pressure of so much demand and activity, we can feel powerless to change the system around us.

But small changes in ourselves can open up a world of possibilities where happiness arises, not from acts of heroism, but from small things done subtly and with mindfulness. Compassion is revealed in the smallest acts.

On some level we already know this; it's as if we sense that the party line is flawed. After all, if mastery of the science and craft of healthcare was enough to create job satisfaction why do we see so much despair and disillusionment among healthcare workers?

Many practitioners blame external factors for their unhappiness, things like overwork, staff shortages, excessive patient demands, bureaucratic systems, funding cutbacks and damaging reorganizations.

Yet in the midst of this chaos, a small number of health professionals go about their work radiating calmness, caring and happiness. Somehow they have learned how to flourish despite the external difficulties.

These gifted practitioners don't neglect their technical skills. In fact they deploy their professional knowledge, experience and skills with remarkable effectiveness. So it's not a case of technical mastery versus humanism in practice. The two go hand in hand.

So it's not a case of technical mastery versus humanism in practice. The two go hand in hand

In the best possible version of ourselves, whether we're a nurse, doctor or therapist, we not only serve patients better but also find greater happiness and contentment in our daily working life.

Kindness is a source of happiness

The researchers in positive psychology have put their microscope on these little building blocks of happiness. One study analyzed the relationship between kindness and happiness in 175 Japanese undergraduate students [3].

Researchers identified three components of kindness:

- Motivation
- Self-recognition
- Behavior

Thus participants were asked to rate themselves with questions like, 'I am always thinking that I wish to be kind and help other people in daily life' and 'I do kind things and help others everyday'.

They measured happiness by asking participants to describe events that produced strong emotions during the last three weeks. Up to five happy events and five unhappy events could be described, and subsequently rated.

Results showed that happy people scored higher on all three components of kindness. They were more strongly motivated to be kind, performed more kind acts, and had more kind thoughts. They also had more happy memories of daily life and felt a greater sense of gratitude.

But which comes first? Are happier people naturally more kind, or does a deliberate focus on kindness lead to happiness?

In the real world, it's been shown that very brief training programs in kindness or appreciation can generate measurable changes in brain and immune function and increase resilience and wellbeing.

In a controlled trial of undergraduate students, researchers examined the impact of a 'Counting Kindness' intervention [3]. Each day for a week, participants were asked to become more aware of their own kind behavior towards other people and to report the daily number of these acts.

While happiness levels in the control group of students didn't change, those in the Counting Kindness group increased significantly. Moreover, the subjects that showed the largest increases in happiness became more kind and grateful, in response to the intervention, compared to those who showed only small changes in happiness.

It seems that a deliberate focus on kindness results in an increase in happiness and a heightened sense of gratitude when on the receiving end of kindness. Increased happiness then motivates more acts of kindness in a virtuous cycle of reinforcement.

Small changes have a big impact on our lives

The research on positive psychology repeats this message: small interventions can make a significant difference to peoples' lives.

One study examined the effect of a few minutes of loving-kindness meditation. Participants were asked to imagine two loved ones standing to either side of the subject and sending their love. After four minutes, subjects were told to open their eyes and redirect these feelings of love and compassion toward the photograph of a neutral stranger appearing in the center of the screen. They also repeated a series of phrases designed to bring attention to the other, and to wish them health, happiness, and wellbeing.

The result was an increased feeling of social connection and positivity towards strangers, revealed both in explicit feelings and subconscious responses such as non-verbal signs [4].

Martin Seligman and colleagues showed that simple exercises, delivered on-line and practiced for just a week, could make a lasting difference to happiness [5]:

Small interventions can make a very significant difference to peoples' lives

One exercise was called 'Three Good Things in Life'. Participants were asked to write down three things that went well each day, and their causes, every night for one week. In addition, they were asked to provide an explanation for each good thing. Follow-up studies showed participants had increased happiness and decreased depressive symptoms for six months after the simple exercise.

In a second experiment they showed that writing and personally delivering one letter of gratitude to someone who had been especially kind, caused large positive changes for a month afterwards.

Focusing on strengths is a third way to improve happiness and guard against depression. Participants took an on-line inventory of character strengths (authentichappiness.org) and practiced using one of their top-five strengths in a new and different way each day for a week. Results were still positive six months on.

Appreciation and gratitude

Appreciation and gratitude are important resources in the toolkit of happy people.

In one study, self-rated 'happy' and 'unhappy' participants recalled and listed observations from one day of their lives that they either appreciated or found frustrating [6]. Happier individuals reported greater sensitivity to reward, greater appreciation in general, and greater appreciation for their memory of events.

There's also increasing evidence that gratitude might even serve as an antidote to materialism.

In a comprehensive review of the research on gratitude, Polak found that individuals who focus on the acquisition of material objects exhibit reduced life satisfaction, diminished levels of happiness, and higher levels of depressive symptoms [7]. In addition to being less satisfied with life as a whole, materialistic people also tend to be less satisfied with other aspects of their lives such as their standard of living, their family life, and the amounts of fun and enjoyment they experience.

Polack then quoted evidence suggesting the positive effects of gratitude could counter materialism:

- Gratitude correlates with positive emotionality, vitality, happiness, satisfaction with life, hope, and optimism
- A tendency to gratitude reduces symptoms of depression and anxiety
- Grateful people have a more positive affect towards neutral words and stimuli and they have more happy memories
- Gratitude motivates people to be more pro-social and generous (as rated by others)
- Gratitude increases trust

Polack concluded that prioritizing material wealth over other values was a significant social problem. By increasing satisfaction with life, raising people's sense of security, and giving them the distinct sense that other people care about them, gratitude might help to alleviate materialistic striving and its negative effects.

As working conditions in healthcare deteriorate, I see many health professionals attempting to find satisfaction and happiness through the pursuit of material wealth. I believe this has the potential to be a misguided and ultimately harmful practice, both for their own happiness and wellbeing, and for the survival of healthcare.

One of the most dramatic turning points in our lives can come when we turn our back on excessive material wealth and choose to lead a simpler life. There's nothing stopping us other than our own fears and insecurities.

Many of the happiest doctors I know are grateful to work for nothing.

One of my anesthesiology colleagues from New Zealand travelled to Nepal, spent nine months at his own expense learning to speak the language like a native, then worked for two years in a remote mountain hospital.

What was his pay? Daily meals and a roof over his head.

Similarly when Ariely studied the motivations for paid and unpaid work he discovered that while people would turn down work they perceived as poorly paid – and be insulted by the offer – they were happy to do the same work for nothing, and in many cases would do a better job than if they were being paid [1].

Research has shown by building positivity and gratitude, an array of coping strategies are strengthened [8]:

- Mindfulness – the ability to direct attention in positive ways
- Seeking emotional support from others
- Asking for practical help
- Positive reinterpretation of the challenging situation
- Active coping by addressing the problems at hand
- Using planning more effectively

Moreover, avoidance strategies – disengagement, denial, substance use, and self-blame – are used less often.

In a similar vein, research on character strengths predictive of life satisfaction identifies five strengths that are consistently and robustly associated: hope, zest, gratitude, love, and curiosity [9].

Building the inner resources for compassion

When we are faced with challenging or distressing situations in our clinical work, our response is the result of a battle between two independent motivational systems that regulate our behavior.

As I described in chapter 4, *Mind How You Care*, one system regulates approach behavior to attain rewards and goals – the approach system. The other system regulates withdrawal and/or inhibition of behavior in response to threat and punishment – the withdrawal system.

This internal battle is especially important in the response to patients' or our own distress. Empathy makes us sensitive to other's suffering and we experience emotions in sympathy – including pain, anxiety, sadness, grief and even horror.

At that crucial juncture, how are we going to behave? Which motivation system will win? Do we withdraw into clinical detachment, or can we stay with the feelings and allow compassion to guide an openhearted approach to the suffering patient?

The regular practice of kindness, gratitude, love and appreciation all help us strengthen the positive centers in our brain so that the approach motivation wins; we can tolerate the distress, show compassion and stay with the patient. The reward is further activation of positive emotional circuits, rather than a retreat into fear and defensiveness.

Structural changes are wired into the brain with repeated practice of these skills. We grow new synaptic connections, strengthen existing ones and even create entirely new neurons to enlarge the positive centers of our brain when we practice kindness.

This brain plasticity is a recent finding. When I went to medical school in the 1980s we were taught the number of neurons in the brain steadily declined during life and that new neurons couldn't be created. Now we know that even the adult brain has astonishing plasticity throughout life [10].

Increasing creativity and social contribution

And as we deliberately choose to focus attention on positive thoughts and emotions, something remarkable happens to our perception, which Frederickson calls the broaden-and-build phenomenon [11].

When our brain is in a positive frame of mind, our perceptual field expands. We literally see more of the world around us, sense greater possibilities, our imagination and creativity are fired up, and we connect more deeply to the people around us. Our capacity for social contribution is enhanced.

It's almost as if those who are flourishing in positivity have been vaccinated against unhappiness. While bad things still happen in the lives of people flourishing in positivity, their reactions are out of the ordinary.

They see the good in the bad. They more easily understand and forgive those who have transgressed against them.

Their good humor and calm nature are not easily disturbed. They don't take things so personally. They are much less likely to get angry. And no matter how bad the situation they rarely feel like helpless victims, they find a way to respond with positivity.

Sometimes the happy people in the world are derisively called 'Pollyanna', referring to the over-optimistic and pathologically cheerful heroine of a children's book. But healthcare is a serious business, lives are at risk, and people suffer. So it's understandable if healthcare tends to be filled with negative thinking and there is justifiable suspicion of those who are over-cheerful.

To casual observers it might seem that over-happy people working in healthcare fail to appreciate suffering or tragedy.

Happy people don't take problems seriously, and have only a superficial connection to patients. But the opposite is true of those who find the greatest happiness in healthcare.

People in a positive state have heightened perception and notice more patient cues. Conversely, people who stuck in problem identification and solving mode – negative thinking – lose their perceptual ability and start to become detached from those around them.

This is one of the paradoxes: the happiest healthcare workers feel the pain of their patients more than average; they are the most empathetic. They care deeply and actually have heightened sensitivity.

Their job satisfaction comes from a deep connection with their patients as admirable and courageous human beings. They regard their work as a privilege. Rather than resenting demands made upon them, they see each as an opportunity for positive and satisfying interaction.

While they witness tragedy and share tears with patients and family members, the strength of their compassion and caring is such that they derive enormous satisfaction from the difference that their caring made to someone's suffering, pain or loss.

Those who have found happiness and contentment in healthcare are also kinder to themselves. They exercise self-compassion. They are comfortable with the idea that human beings are flawed, vulnerable and sometimes broken.

When they don't judge themselves so harshly, they are kinder about the difficulties of others.

Fulfilling your ideals and aspirations

People enter the health professions with a deep desire to care; yet too often their caring and humanity is suppressed by the culture of the institutions in which they find themselves immersed. But when a window of opportunity arises, that caring and compassion is waiting to flourish anew.

You don't need anyone's permission. Nobody can stop you. You have the power to transform your daily work experience, to find joy and satisfaction in your care of patients, and to allow your compassion and caring to rise above the restrictions of institutional rules and practices.

And remember: positivity is contagious! You can help transform the lives of your patients and those who work around you.

Chapter 13

HEARTS IN HEALTHCARE

HEARTS in HEALTHCARE is a worldwide community engaging health professionals, patient and consumer activists, students, managers, teachers, leaders, researchers, lawyers, architects – indeed anyone who wants to work together to help re-humanize healthcare.

I'd like to introduce you to the kind of people who offer inspiration within the movement:

Claire is a physician in the USA, a solo mum with disabled children, who herself had to learn to walk again after a devastating neurological illness. It took doctors nearly two years to diagnose her problem.

Some might become bitter when life delivers so many cruel blows. Claire is one of the people who grow through adversity.

She knows what it is to be broken and she reaches out to help other physicians in need.

She has experienced how cruel the healthcare system can be and her empathy and understanding of patients' suffering is profound.

Claire offered to work for nothing in support of HEARTS in HEALTHCARE; you couldn't find a more passionate advocate.

Helen is an archeologist and mum living in Massachusetts. Her great gift is pulling together fragments of evidence to tell a compelling story.

It's not often that a layperson gets invited to deliver a keynote address at a Harvard Healthcare Quality Improvement Symposium. Helen's address is one of the most electrifying I have heard.

With her sharp powers of observation she describes with horrifying precision the clinical signs of impending shock in her young son. He was the victim of a serious medical error after routine surgery. Calling for help again and again, she witnessed his progressive deterioration over two days, culminating in a cardiac arrest and death. These events occurred in a hospital ward; all her cries of alarm were brushed off.

Helen has forgiven her son's surgeon and she now works with healthcare leaders to strengthen patient safety. She's come to a compassionate understanding of how caring health workers can make mistakes and what it takes to support healing after tragedy.

Andrew is a medical student leader in New Zealand. He knows that his fellow students entered medical school with high ideals of compassionate, patient-centered care. But he's worried that the overwhelming focus on biomedicine and disease processes is robbing students of their humanity. So he's drawing on the power of international medical student associations to support our movement.

When his fellow students voted a lecture on 'compassion' the best of the year, the Faculty took notice. Now they're developing a new curriculum module on empathy.

Seigfried is an architect designing healthcare facilities in Australia. He resigned from a big architectural practice to set up his own consultancy. His passion is designing healthcare facilities to attract and retain health workers. His theory is simple: happy and healthy workers, will care better for patients and be more likely to stay in the healthcare workforce.

Belinda is a nurse in Scotland, one of the inspirational figures behind the Leadership in Compassionate Care project in Edinburgh. One of her projects was exploring the use of Emotional Touch Points in conversations with patients.

The idea is very simple. She has a deck of cards, each card naming an emotion like 'happy' or 'embarrassed' or 'proud' or 'angry' or 'grateful'. In conversations with patients, she asks them to remember moments in their care that had particular emotional significance, good or bad. She then asks the patient to pick the card that best describes their feeling about the moment.

Using that emotion as a starting point, the team can then explore what behaviors of the heath professionals led to that emotion. It gives deep insight into the patient experience of care.

Kathy is a lawyer in San Francisco with a radical concept for her profession: being servants in support of resolution and healing after injury, rather than adversaries. She sees how much suffering is caused when patients injured by medical error have to sue their doctors to get answers. She knows adversarial processes cause much harm to medical professionals too. She's devoted a lifetime to facilitating legal processes of resolution that allow all the parties to come together, seek forgiveness, learn from mistakes, and build a safer system.

Tess is a receptionist in the community medical centre. She noticed that kids of poor families often attended poorly clothed, some didn't even have shoes in winter. So she started up a clothing bank at the clinic. When appointment letters were posted, she'd include a paper slip asking parents to bring donations of clothes or shoes their kids had outgrown. Pretty soon, parents started bring toys too!

Now every kid from a poor family goes home with the present of a toy and maybe some new warm clothes. What used to be a frightening ordeal for the kids – visiting the doctor – turned into a treat.

David is a medical resident, working up acute medical patients in the emergency department. He always goes the extra mile for his patients. One afternoon he had a patient with chest pain, worried about a heart condition. Initial exams were negative but the patient needed a treadmill test. The cardiology department was closing down for the day – nobody to do the test. 'No worries,' said David, 'I'll supervise the test myself.' It kept him late after the end of his shift but it allowed the patient to go home, reassured.

That's just typical of David. He won't hesitate to do some little service for a patient if he can quickly solve a problem or respond to a need.

Michelle is an occupational therapist working with patients who have suffered a stroke. Her department is seriously short-staffed and it's a struggle to meet the basic needs of patients including help with daily activities like eating a meal. Appeals for staffing improvement fell of deaf ears – the budget was blown already.

So how did Michelle respond? Working with a local high school, she built a scheme for student volunteers to visit the hospital ward and help with the daily non-medical needs of patients. The students had a great work experience, which was integrated into their school curriculum. The patients loved the contact with young people and their care was improved. And the School of Occupational Therapy noticed an increase in enrollments.

These are all people who care deeply but for most of their working lives they have felt isolated and alone. They are deeply empathetic to the suffering of patients and feel compelled to respond. But their efforts to provide more responsive, compassionate care have met resistance.

All too often the institutional policies and unwritten rules reward workers' attention to clinical tasks and fast throughput, rather than thoughtful listening, caring and healing. Many health professionals have become cynical and battle-hardened. There are few role models for humane and compassionate care. Peer pressure can be intense. Bullying, abuse and disruptive behavior take their toll.

Those who buck the system and stand up for their patients have a hard time. It takes great courage to openly discuss issues like caring and compassion, personal vulnerability, death and dying.

But these people, with their endless determination, passion and persistence are the vanguards of a positive change sweeping healthcare.

Everyone knows that the relentless pursuit of technology is bankrupting healthcare; that the health demands of an aging population have outstripped available resources; that trying to patch up patients with chronic disease is futile if we don't attend to healthy lifestyles, happiness and well-being. The old system is crumbling and something new must take its place.

If we are determined to lead fundamental change in the healthcare system, what are the best strategies? How can HEARTS in HEALTHCARE catalyze a worldwide movement?

Margaret Wheatley is a leader in strategies for whole-system change and building the capacity of communities to solve their own problems [1,2].

Wheatley says that our existing institutions and leadership models are inadequate for the complex challenges of a deeply interconnected, modern world.

Wheatley would argue that healthcare is a hugely complex, global network that is impossible to manage through top-down leadership.

Take workforce planning, for example. We all know we have a rapidly aging population and the burden of care for chronic diseases is increasing exponentially. A rationally planned and managed healthcare system would ensure we have enough geriatricians to cope with the projected increase in demand, right? That's why we appoint national expert committees to come up with solutions.

Just such a major report is the Institute of Medicine Retooling for an Aging America: Building the Health Care Workforce. The report authors say that in the USA only 7,128 physicians are certified geriatricians [3]. By 2020 the predicted need is 36,000 geriatricians but assuming current rates of growth and attrition, this number will increase to only 7,750 - far short of the total predicted.

In fact, some argue that there could be a net decrease in geriatricians because of the decreasing number of physicians entering training programs as well as the decreasing number of geriatricians who choose to recertify.

So how could a rational system of planning get this so wrong? What really determines the supply of geriatricians?

The answer is doctors work in a global marketplace with infinite choices. After six years at medical school, doctors can choose between a large number of specialties in medicine and surgery.

The attractiveness of any one specialty varies from year to year depending on career prospects, reimbursement systems, working conditions, perceived status, lifestyle options, etc. Even having chosen geriatrics as a career, doctors can make many choices about work location, hours of work, or taking a break to have a family.

If local working conditions deteriorate owing to staffing shortage, system overload, or changing reimbursement rates, then doctors can choose to work in another country.

Economic storms, political crises and even climate change can rapidly turn the tide of physician supply in any given location. A sudden change in one part of the world, such as new rules for professional registration, can tip the balance in far distant lands. All parts of the system are tightly interconnected.

So, no matter how many heavy reports land on the desks of policy makers, our professional, institutional and political leaders are completely unable to solve these complex problems. The problem is not that we have incompetent leaders, but that our models of leadership are completely inadequate in the face of complex, interconnected systems.

Our underlying theories of leadership cast our leaders in the hero mold. Whether we are appointing chief executives or voting for politicians, our working theory is that inspirational leaders will somehow have the right ideas to solve complex problems. It gives an illusion of control. If people just do as they are told and follow the plan, we'll be all right.

And when things start to get out of hand, the response is to impose tighter control and give ever more draconian powers to the leaders.

A good example is the current economic crisis among the debt-ridden nations in Europe. IMF leaders demand of countries like Greece and Spain that government expenditure be savagely cut and taxes raised to reduce debt.

These measures create economic contraction and rising unemployment. Tax revenue falls, the workers go on mass protests, the government falls, and credit rating agencies further downgrade the national status. Cost of borrowing increases and the debt situation worsens.

Often it seems that every action taken by the leaders only makes the situation worse. Then when everything turns to custard, what do we do? We sack the elected leaders and appoint technocrats who are supposed to have the answers!

Attempts to reform healthcare in the USA have focused on insurance systems, reimbursement rates, policy exclusions and cost control – sounds familiar? But these top-down systems of change will never work in the face of complexity.

Workforce planning is just one tiny example of the complexity and global interdependence in healthcare. If you examine any aspect of the system you will find similarly uncontrollable dynamics.

All our existing institutions, whether they are health, education, or even governments – are struggling to address the complexity and speed of change.

Wheatley promotes a different model of leadership, to suit the complexities of the modern world. She talks about leaders as 'hosts' rather than 'heroes' [4]. What does she mean?

Whole-system change occurs, argues Wheatley, in a natural process of emergence [5]. As different ideas start to connect up across global networks, the system can reach a tipping point where a major shift suddenly occurs.

Examples in the political system include the fall of the Berlin Wall that so powerfully symbolized the collapse of the Soviet empire. More recently, the spread of the democratic revolution in North Africa and the Middle East is an example of how people mobilized through social networks can overthrow repressive regimes.

This process of change occurs in four stages:

1. Isolated pioneers struggling alone
2. Networks linking together, discovering shared meaning and purpose
3. Communities of practice sharing learning and developing new practices together
4. Systems of influence where the new practices become the norm

The new breed of leaders doesn't pretend to know the answers to complex problems. But they have the deepest faith in the creative capacity of people to work together and allow new and surprising solutions to emerge from within complexity.

The new role of the leader is to nourish the conversations, to connect together the pioneers, to foster communities of practice, and to promote the spread of good ideas. The leader is the host not the hero.

HEARTS in HEALTHCARE is specifically designed to follow these principles.

We have no idea how or where the transformation of healthcare will take place or what are the best strategies to strengthen caring and compassion in whole systems. But we do know that healthcare is full of incredibly passionate, smart, and hard working individuals who know how to solve little bits of the puzzle.

The pioneers in this change are the kind of people I mentioned at the beginning of the chapter. Some have reached positions of influence, after many years of struggle, but most are just trying to do the best job they can in difficult circumstances.

Often they have come up with creative solutions but they have no idea that their work has broader significance. They are too humble to imagine that others facing the same problems would value their ideas.

Often these pioneers feel deeply isolated. Their values and ideals are at odds with the prevailing culture but they persist in their efforts because they witness so much unnecessary suffering and they know the system could work better. Good ideas just have to fall on fertile ground. Where you work, it might not be the right time to introduce a new idea. In another place, it might flourish.

The best leaders call from the heart. They reach within themselves to find authentic values and principles that serve as a common calling, a means to bind together a community with shared purpose.

Rachel Naomi Remen and colleagues in the Institute for the Study of Health and Illness (ISHI) at Commonweal developed a program for undergraduates students called The Healers' Art, now offered in many medical schools around the world [6]. They talk about authentic community as an educational strategy for advancing professionalism.

The course provides a safe community in which students can legitimize the humanistic elements of professionalism and gain insights into the relationship between physicians and patients. This fifteen-hour course is a tiny island of hope in a sea of impersonalized biomedicine.

Similar outreach programs from ISHI support small groups of physicians to form story-telling and discussion groups for Finding Meaning in Medicine [7]. They remark, "It has been ISHI's experience that physicians themselves are presently far more interested in such programs of mutual support than are their employers."

These pioneering efforts are gradually spreading but nowhere have I found a community that welcomes all different kinds of health professionals – not just doctors – to join together with patient activists and others who are passionate about re-humanizing healthcare.

So HEARTS in HEALTHCARE is designed to be a safe haven, a place where the people who care the most can come together in authentic community and find their values and ideals legitimized and supported.

Too much of healthcare is corrupted with competition, greed and moneymaking. In some places patients have become 'profit centers' and practice is shaped according to financial return, rather than what is best for the patient.

HEARTS in HEALTHCARE is based on the values of caring and compassion, mutual support, and a humble approach to learning and wisdom. We know that the deepest satisfaction and meaning in life arises in the service to others.

So the first job of HEARTS in HEALTHCARE is to provide mutual support and encouragement to pioneers who have been struggling alone. We are hosting an on-line community of like-minded individuals from many different backgrounds, one that provides encouragement, shared learning, inspiration and friendship.

The second role of HEARTS in HEALTHCARE is to build the capacity of our members to make a positive contribution – through strengthening their happiness, wellbeing and resilience. Positivity is infectious. Not only can members support each other to grow and develop, they'll also start teaching these skills to their patients.

The third role of HEARTS in HEALTHCARE is to foster communities of practice, to promote the best ideas and encourage small groups in many different locations to work together and experiment with new practices. Like-minded groups will start to connect and share ideas.

The fourth role of HEARTS in HEALTHCARE is to provide a mechanism to highlight the best ideas, the most effective solutions, the greatest teachers, and most inspirational leaders. This is a natural process of evolution driven by the social networks within the community. The direction of the community is driven entirely by the members – we have no idea who or what is going to emerge.

The fifth role of HEARTS in HEALTHCARE is to influence the system from within by walking the talk. We will not try to persuade authority figures or impose change but we'll find a thousand ways to support those leaders who want to work in a different way. And we'll celebrate success.

Although we are clear about our different roles in hosting the community, we don't know how best to support those functions. Yet again, we are confident the members of our community will come up with the best ideas to work together and take us forward.

The inspiring stories of personal transformation, and the scientific evidence presented in this book, lead us to believe that re-connecting to the heart of your practice is good for your health, wellbeing and happiness. In a major research collaboration with Dr Martin Seligman, the founding father of positive psychology, we aim to prove that hypothesis.

Members of the HEARTS in HEALTHCARE community will be invited to participate in longitudinal studies of their happiness, compassionate caring, work satisfaction, and meaning in life. Using scientifically validated, on-line questionnaires, we'll ask our members to complete a self-assessment on first registration and then repeat the measures each year.

Engaging with our community, learning how to strengthen your heart, choosing to love your work, gaining skills for compassionate caring, and becoming part of a global movement to re-humanize healthcare may be the best investment in your health and wellbeing that you ever make!

There are 60 million health professionals in the world. If only a small percent are ready for this change that's enough to create a powerful, global network.

We know from history that motivated health professionals, working together can change the course of history.

Founded in 1980, International Physicians for the Prevention of Nuclear War (ippnw.org) was an inspiration born of the Cold War [8].

With the world divided into two militarized camps poised on the brink of nuclear war, a small group of Soviet and American doctors founded an international movement, believing their shared concern for humanity overcame ideological differences.

Co-founders Drs. Bernard Lown, Jim Muller, Eric Chivian and Herb Abrams of the US and Drs. Evgueni Chazov, Mikhail Kuzin and Leonid Ilyin of the Soviet Union, organized a team to conduct meticulous scientific research on the effects of the atomic bombs dropped on Hiroshima and Nagasaki.

Within five years, IPPNW had expanded to a network of 150,000 physicians who sounded a medical warning to humanity: that nuclear war would be the final epidemic; that there would be no cure and no meaningful medical response. Their message reached millions of people around the world.

In 1985, at the height of the Cold War, IPPNW won the Nobel Peace Prize. Dr Lown traveled to Moscow and was one of the first westerners to meet Gorbachev, the Soviet leader. They talked for three hours.

Following this historic meeting, Gorbachev decided to begin a process of unilateral disarmament. The world pulled back from the brink of nuclear catastrophe.

Incredibly, this global network of physicians came into being before the days of the Internet.

Imagine the capacity we now have to create a truly global movement to re-humanize healthcare and reduce suffering in the world.

Join us today at HEARTSinHEALTHCARE.com

Chapter 14

MY STORY: REBEL WITH A GOOD CAUSE

Sitting in a huge lecture theatre at Bristol medical school in 1980, on the first day of term, I wondered what fate awaited me. As one of only six mature students among hundreds of young school leavers, I felt out of place.

Just getting to medical school was the realization of a hard-won ambition. I'd completed an engineering degree at Cambridge and worked for three years in the highest-paid job I could find – international oil exploration – to fund my studies.

Our seismic exploration crew was paid vast sums of money for each day of survey data. At age twenty-two, I was earning more than my father, a senior medical specialist. Working in the Niger Delta of West Africa, we lived in a savage environment far from civilization. On a regular basis we dealt with thievery, corruption, tribal disputes, murder, black magic, and tropical diseases.

The work was dangerous: I was once held up at gunpoint, twice nearly drowned in huge surf, narrowly avoided being blown up by dynamite, and on one dreadful day found myself at the centre of a pitched battle where limbs were hacked off with machetes.

A timely vacancy in the New Zealand seismic crew sent me briefly to New Plymouth in 1979. Within a month of arriving, I met my wife Meredith. We have now been together thirty-three years and have three beautiful daughters and two grandchildren.

Most of my oil exploration colleagues survived the brutality of the job for only two or three years before quitting with a small fortune. In three years I saved enough for a deposit on a small home, a new car, and funds to pay the fees for the many years of medical school.

My life experience and confidence proved to be a source of trouble in the years ahead. The rules for success in the British medical establishment were very clear: work all hours, don't rock the boat, and never challenge your seniors. I had trouble with these rules.

My father was an eye surgeon who turned down offers of lucrative private practice because he believed medicine and business didn't mix well and that clinical decisions should be based only on the patient's best interest. I'd chosen medicine because, like my father, I wanted to serve people in an honorable profession.

As I rose up the ranks of medical practice, I applied my engineering and system knowledge to the human dynamics within hospitals – and became fascinated by the interaction of different professional groups working together for patient care.

The results of my analysis were discouraging. In what should have been caring and compassionate organizations I found widespread bullying, powerful hierarchies, professional rivalries, and dehumanizing practices. The poor patients were at the bottom of the pile and were largely powerless and vulnerable.

I soon found myself acting as the defender of the sick and vulnerable. In my first internship I decided my role was as ambassador for my patients. I established friendly, diplomatic relations with the key people in different departments, like the clerk who scheduled x-rays, to ensure my patients got the best possible service.

The hospital work hours were insane. My longest stretch was fourteen days and nights of continuous duty except for three individual nights when I was allowed to leave the hospital and see my wife and children.

The long hours did allow me to get to know my patients intimately. Many were bewildered, fearful and rendered completely helpless by the institutional practices and professional norms of behavior.

While working as a junior resident, I wrote and published a book, *OPERATION! A Handbook for Surgical Patients*. It was my attempt to give patients some power back in the system, and to answer their many questions.

Our happy home was a precious refuge from the stresses of hospital life and I feel sure that Meredith's love and understanding allowed me to retain some humanity and compassion in my patient care. She also taught me to touch and show tenderness – qualities missing in my upbringing.

Two years into my practice I began training in anesthesia. The early days were terrifying, with the awful potential to make a mistake and kill a patient within minutes. In my first training post I was grateful for the close supervision and support of my seniors.

Anesthesiologists are often pioneers for adopting systematic approaches to patient safety, seeking inspiration from high-reliability industries like aviation. Anesthesia was the first to use anonymous incident reporting and analysis of near-miss incidents to uncover system failures that put patients at risk. I took a keen interest in patient safety, bolstered by my engineering background.

Imagining patient safety to be a largely scientific and technical issue, I was surprised to discover system failures involved many human factors and moral conflicts. Confidential enquiries into patient deaths had highlighted poor supervision of inexperienced trainees was a major risk factor for patient injury or death, particularly for high-risk emergency cases done outside normal working hours.

This was just the situation I found myself in when I joined the anesthesia residency program at the large teaching hospital.

The chairman of the department of anesthesia called a meeting of trainees and said, 'We're here to support you. I'm going to go round the whole room and ask each of you individually if you have any concerns or worries.'

The body language was instructive. Everyone looked at the floor and avoided eye contact with the chairman. I was two-thirds of the way around the circle and every person before me denied any issues or worries.

'Robin?' he asked.

Taking a deep breath I lifted my eyes and offered a provocative challenge.

'Yes, I'm very concerned about patient safety in the maternity department after hours. Twice in the last two weeks, I have almost failed to intubate an obese patient having an emergency cesarean section. I'd like to know why there is no anesthesia technician to assist the most junior trainees doing high-risk cases in the night?'

Of course senior anesthesiologists always had a skilled anesthetic nurse or technician to help them with routine, day-time cases but in the maternity department at night, the anesthetic trainees had only midwives to assist, who were unskilled in the specialist tasks of the anesthetic procedure.

My challenge caused a deathly hush in the room and everyone held their breath. The Chairman answered coldly, 'Well of course Robin, you've had these problems and nobody else seems to be concerned about this. Maybe you should be reflecting on your own practice?'

He continued smoothly, 'I'm sure in the next couple of years when we build the new hospital, we should be able to provide some cross-cover for assistance at night.'

I became reckless in my outrage, protesting, 'To be perfectly frank, if I was chairman of the department I would ensure there was skilled assistance available for trainees at nighttime by next Monday, not in two years' time! Do we have to wait for a mother to die before we do anything else about this?'

There were gasps around the room. I was committing professional suicide but I hadn't finished this rebellion.

Some months later the Royal College of Anaesthetists sent inspectors to interview residents. I gave candid accounts of the dangers posed by lack of supervision for the trainees. Nothing came of my concerns; I soon discovered that several of my consultants were members of the College Council.

I appealed to the committee of the Regional Training Scheme, which was stacked with representatives from my own hospital.

But the Old Boys' Network was closing ranks: Youngson was clearly a troublemaker.

A better life in New Zealand

Soon after completing my anesthesia fellowship in England, we had decided to return to New Zealand permanently. We sold our home, put all of our belongings in a shipping container, and burnt our bridges.

The medical culture in the UK was increasingly oppressive and I had already damaged my career prospects. Soon after, the British medical establishment was rocked by huge scandal: incompetent cardiac surgeons at Bristol Royal Infirmary had caused the deaths of more than a hundred babies and small children. The whistleblower, an anesthesiologist, lost his job and had to flee the country.

I signed up for the Auckland anesthesia training scheme, committing myself to sitting the Australasian anesthesia fellowship exam.

In 1994, I was appointed as a specialist anesthesiologist at Auckland Public Hospital, the biggest teaching hospital in New Zealand. Meredith and I had made a major investment in family life in Auckland, we'd built a home, our girls were settled in their schools, and Meredith was immersed in the local community.

An introduction to patient-centered redesign

Like most big hospitals at the time, Auckland Hospital had a growing problem in the surgical department: the patients coming for surgery were getting steadily older and sicker.

The spiraling risks caused tension between surgeons and anesthesiologists. Surgeons wanted a smooth operating schedule but anesthesiologist were canceling cases at short notice because patients' medical conditions had not been adequately treated, escalating the risk of anesthesia and surgery.

I knew many patient care problems were caused by system failures. My engineering mind was beginning to see possibilities for a radical process redesign, centered on the needs of patients.

When I applied for the job at Auckland Hospital, I submitted with my CV a business plan for a systematic overhaul of the pre-operative process.

This entrepreneurial initiative astonished and impressed the appointment committee. The government was putting extreme pressure on the health boards to become more efficient and financially accountable so my 'business-like' approach found favor.

Not only did I win the job but the terms of my appointment were unusual: I was given a full salary to work half-time in the operating rooms and half-time leading patient process redesign.

A year later I published our first report. A talented multidisciplinary team had trialed a radical redesign of the pre-operative process and we had the data to prove the benefits.

Patient cancellations had been eliminated, the surgical lists ran like clockwork, there were fewer critical incidents and complications, patient satisfaction was up, we eliminated many unnecessary activities, and substantially cut costs.

I was even invited to present our findings to the Minister of Health and found myself on a conference discussion panel sandwiched between the Minister and the President of the College of Surgeons. This was giddy fame for a newly appointed specialist.

The celebrations were short-lived. Even though we had won over the surgeons and anesthesiologists, hospital management opposed the introduction of the new streamlined care pathway.

It gradually dawned the problem was higher up the management hierarchy. It was a painful lesson in the complexities of healthcare politics. Perverse incentives prevented a change for the better.

I knew many other clinical leaders around the country who had great ideas for better care. But they were all feeling isolated and marginalized. So I took action. In 1998 I set up an incorporated society, the Clinical Leaders' Association of New Zealand (CLANZ).

The Minister of Health, impressed with our initiative and the success of our first gathering, gave us a little seed funding. First we researched the learning needs of clinicians rising into leadership roles.

Armed with this report, I went back to see the Minister. After a twenty minute meeting, I secured agreement for half a million dollars funding for CLANZ.

The next decade was one of tumultuous change in healthcare. I was appointed to a national committee advising the government on healthcare quality and safety. I subsequently found myself working with the World Health Organizations on strategies for patient safety, and people at the center of healthcare.

In 2000, I left my job at the big teaching hospital to join an inspirational leadership team designing and building a new hospital within my own, underprivileged community. For many years I worked part-time in anesthesia and part-time in leadership roles.

Through CLANZ, I was directly involved in developing a multimedia learning resource for health professionals, illustrating the patients' experience of care. Their dramatized, first hand accounts of what it's like to be a patient proved to be a real eye-opener for health professionals.

I used these videos in dozens of workshops with mixed groups of health professionals and learned from workshop participants that the problems patients described were universal.

I was outspoken about patient safety, taking my campaigns to the media. We did some pioneering work on open disclosure and apology after medical error. We also showed that courageous and skillful approaches to healing inter-professional conflicts could help transform clinical services.

However, working with the national committee, the Ministry of Health, and the politicians was for me a bizarre experience. I learned that authority systems were very handicapped in dealing with the natural complexity of the system.

The government funding for CLANZ was contingent on agreeing a concrete set of contract deliverables – which didn't align with our vision of a dynamic network of inspired clinical leaders. Diverted from our purpose, we began to neglect our members. We fulfilled our Ministry contracts but funding was pulled and the network died.

Healthcare reform gets personal

I have long been passionate about patient-centered care but it was the experience of our teenage daughter Chloe that showed us how hospital systems can be lacking in basic care and compassion.

Following a serious car crash in 2004, Chloe spent a hundred days in hospital in spinal traction with a broken neck.

She has recovered fully. The technical quality of her clinical care was generally good and we are deeply grateful to the many expert practitioners who helped her mend and recover.

However, the gross neglect of her basic human needs, such as her psychological wellbeing, the provision of disability aids, or getting the food she needed for healing, was profoundly shocking.

Moreover, although I had previously been a senior specialist in this hospital, and a member of the executive team, I found myself powerless to address many of the failings.

One day she was left in excruciating pain for many hours although the plan for her pain relief was carefully documented in her records and the medications needed were available on the ward. The system of care failed to join the dots.

When we asked, begged and pleaded with the ward staff to take the next simple step for pain relief, they said they weren't familiar with the treatment. As the situation escalated, what we witnessed was a kind of learned helplessness.

The nurses were clearly distressed with Chloe's suffering but felt unable to act and they began to hide from us. As we escalated the problem to more senior people in the hierarchy, the response became callous and uncaring. We were blamed for causing a fuss and "making the nurses feel threatened". In the meantime, Chloe was still weeping in pain.

We quickly learned to be deeply circumspect in the ways in which we interacted with the hospital staff, on whose goodwill and care depended the survival of our daughter. We were endlessly polite, friendly, appreciative and affirming.

As we tested the system, we came to understand the profound lack of caring and compassion at the system level, even though individual health professionals did their best.

Through this experience and many others in various leadership roles I came to appreciate that we could hardly expect nurses and doctors to show compassion unless the system itself treated them with humanity and compassion – far from the norm in today's stressed healthcare institutions.

The question is how do we change the system? How do we re-humanize healthcare and liberate caring and compassion?

In New Zealand there is a legal Code of Rights for Health & Disability Consumers, and an independent Commissioner to investigate complaints. We felt sure that Chloe's care had neglected many of her legal rights. We made a complaint to the Commission on her behalf, saying we were satisfied with the clinical treatment but had profound concerns about the neglect of her basic needs. We hoped to create a precedent.

Sadly, we discovered that the investigation of a complaint is largely based on the hospital records, which are almost completely silent on the matters that concerned us so gravely. The voices missing from the clinical record are those of the patient and family.

On the basis of the evidence available, the Commissioner felt unable to record a breach of rights, although he raised many serious concerns in his letter to the chief executive of the health board.

If such a blatant disregard of human needs was not sufficient to trigger a breach of rights, we reasoned, then the Code of Rights needed to be strengthened. We mounted a national campaign add a new right to the Code, "The right to be treated with compassion."

To mount such a campaign we needed a new vehicle for change and the ability to speak with independence. So, having learned the potential dangers of government funding, we founded the Compassion in Healthcare Charitable Trust in 2006, and began fundraising.

We also took many of the lessons of Chloe's experience to design better care processes and policies for our new community hospital.

We radically changed our visitor policy so that every patient was entitled to nominate a family member as a 'Care Partner'.

The care partner was given a temporary name badge and was engaged as part of the clinical team, entitled to be present at any time, day or night.

The Compassion in Healthcare Trust was founded on a vision of an inspiring demonstration hospital, where caring and compassion would flourish.

There was strong support from my hospital leadership team and the local community raised money in support of the cause, with the support of the hospital foundation. But in the end, we were subject to the goodwill and support of people who had other agendas.

A new chief executive was appointed at the health board and the local hospital leaders all lost their jobs in a management restructure.

My clinical leadership role was abolished and I lost half my income. The executive director of the hospital foundation was left without support and quit her job. The Compassion in Healthcare Trust was wound down.

I finally walked away from my anesthesia job in 2011. It was too dispiriting to continue to work in a hospital where so much good was being eroded and I wanted to devote more of my time and energy to global efforts to re-humanize healthcare.

As a clinician I still witness every day the unnecessary suffering, to both patients and health professionals, caused by inhumane and unsafe care systems. I am deeply motivated to address these problems but I have to reflect on whether my actions achieve their purpose. Am I part of the problem?

Stepping away from conflict

In the end, I sensed my continued presence in the hospital merely served to sustain conflict. I was getting in the way of other positive changes. I had two farewell dinners and was deeply touched by the reminders of how much we had achieved together and expressions of regret that I was leaving.

Above all, I had learned that the culture of a hospital can be changed for the better quite quickly. Many of our gains in supporting compassionate caring, and creating a healthy and safe working environment for the health workers, have persisted – they are woven into the fabric of the institution.

Both CLANZ and the Compassion in Healthcare Trust did a huge amount of work over ten years. Very dedicated individuals served as board directors or trustees and, if nothing else, we succeeded in raising awareness of important issues. It's easy to forget in the late 1990's issues such as patient safety, clinical leadership, and compassion in healthcare were really beneath the political radar.

After fifteen years of determined efforts to improve patient care I no longer try to persuade people to alter their ways. People naturally resist change. When you push, persuade, argue and even threaten you can achieve change but is it sustainable? Will the system slip back to its previous state the moment you take the pressure off?

Change will only be sustainable if it makes life better or easier for people. Of course the benefits may not initially be obvious, or they may be recognized by only a few – the so-called 'early adopters' of any change that sweeps the world.

For health professionals, the old equation for happiness doesn't work any more: study hard, gain specialized qualifications, develop your expertise, raise your status and self-esteem, earn a good income – and you should have a happy and rewarding career.

Instead, we have epidemic levels of stress, unhappiness and burnout among health professionals. A new equation of benefits is required.

The Compassion in Healthcare Trust identified a good cause and many people wanted to support us, but it didn't adequately identify how we could transform the lives of our supporters while at the same time achieving our goals of re-humanizing healthcare.

I hope and believe that with HEARTS in HEALTHCARE we have that equation right.

The evidence is compelling: reconnecting to the heart of your practice, learning compassionate caring, and liberating your practice from organizational restrictions is the way to happiness and wellbeing.

It's also how we will transform healthcare.

So rather than trying to persuade, we'll just offer this opportunity to those who are ready and willing. The rest will come to us in time. Our early adopters will become the evangelists that spread the word and encourage the next wave of supporters.

I have stepped away from all authority roles and I now devote my time and energy to this grassroots social movement within healthcare. I don't ignore authority figures; I just wait for them to show interest.

In New Zealand, there are twenty district health boards each with a chief executive. Nineteen of them don't currently have caring and compassion as a strategic priority. One does. One says, "This is what we are here for". She's strongly supporting a pilot trial of HEARTS in HEALTHCARE in her hospital.

In our new strategy, one is enough.

I was a medical laboratory technician in New Plymouth when I met the young engineer who worked for a British oil exploration company. While I liked Robin immediately I really became interested in getting to know him better when he told me of his aspirations to go to medical school.

That he was prepared to work in some pretty uncomfortable and perilous situations to fund himself through medical school, was an impressive testament to both his character and his commitment.

At that time I saw medicine as a profession that cared deeply about people and easing suffering in the world; values that strongly resonated with me, and Robin apparently viewed it the same way.

As his wife, I watched Robin go through the brutalizing process of Med School in the UK with a mixture of admiration and horror.

I still remember being sickened by the callousness of a surgical consultant who regaled us at a dinner party with stories of the heroic surgical procedures he carried out, without once referring to a patient as a whole person, or reflecting on the psychological or emotional effects those patients endured in order to live.

After one particularly horrific weekend when a number of Robin's patients died and he was first in line to deal with the patients and then their devastated families, Robin arrived home on his bicycle looking anguished and desperately upset. He crumpled into my arms and wept, while gradually telling me all that had happened that weekend. I wept too, and wondered at a system that could expose a young adult to this trauma without any support or counseling.

And as we wept, I fervently hoped and prayed that he would never stop feeling like this; that he would never become clinically detached from the pain and suffering of other human beings the way so many of his colleagues seemed to.

And although he has been through some difficult times, and has felt pretty frustrated and grumpy with both staff and patients occasionally, I know that he has never stopped being the kind, caring compassionate man who made such a commitment to medicine over 30 years ago.

- Meredith Youngson 2012

NOTES TO THE CHAPTERS

Chapter 1 Notes

1. Rosenstein, A.H., Disruptive physician behavior. Strategies for addressing the cause and effect. Healthcare executive, 2011. 26(1): p. 78-9.

2. Maben, J., S. Latter, and J.M. Clark, The sustainability of ideals, values and the nursing mandate: evidence from a longitudinal qualitative study. Nursing Inquiry, 2007. 14(2): p. 99-113.

3. Merritt Hawkins & Associates, The Physicians' Perspective: Medical Practice in 2008, The Physicians' Foundation: USA.

4. Rosenstein, A.H. and M. O'Daniel, Disruptive behavior and clinical outcomes: perceptions of nurses and physicians. The American journal of nursing, 2005. 105(1): p. 54-64.

5. Sweet, G.S. and H.J. Wilson, A patient's experience of ward rounds. Patient Education and Counseling, 2010. In press.

6. Veenhoven, R., Healthy happiness: effects of happiness on physical health and the consequences for preventive health care. Journal of Happiness Studies, 2008. 9(3): p. 449-469.

7. Gouin, J.P. and J.K. Kiecolt-Glaser, The impact of psychological stress on wound healing: methods and mechanisms. Immunology and allergy clinics of North America, 2011. 31(1): p. 81-93.

8. Godbout, J.P. and R. Glaser, Stress-induced immune dysregulation: implications for wound healing, infectious disease and cancer. Journal of neuroimmune pharmacology : the official journal of the Society on Neuroimmune Pharmacology, 2006. 1(4): p. 421-7.

9. Kivimaki, M., et al., Sickness absence in hospital physicians: 2 year follow up study on determinants. Occupational and Environmental Medicine, 2001. 58(6): p. 361-366.

10. Sweeney, K., L. Toy, and J. Cornwell, A patient's journey: Mesothelioma. BMJ, 2009. 339: p. 511-514.

11. Menzies, I., A case study in the functioning of social systems as a defence against anxiety. Human Relations, 1960. 13: p. 95-121.

12. Treadway, K. and N. Chatterjee, Into the Water — The Clinical Clerkships. The New England Journal of Medicine, 2011. 364;13: p. 1190-1193.

13. Seligman, M.E.P., Learned optimism. 1990, New York, N.Y.: Pocket Books. 319 p.

14. Seligman, M.E.P., Positive Health. Applied Psychology: An International ReviewN, 2008. 57: p. 3-18.

15. Boersma E, M.A., Deckers JW, Simoons ML. , Early thrombolytic treatment in acute myocardial infarction: reappraisal of the golden hour. Lancet, 1996. 348: p. 771-75.

16. Peterson, C.S., M., Character Strengths and Virtues: A Handbook and Classification. 2004, Washington, DC: American Psychological Association / Oxford University Press.

17. Fredrickson, B., Positivity : groundbreaking research to release your inner optimist and thrive. 2010, Richmond: Oneworld.

18. Fredrickson, B., et al., Open hearts build lives: Positive emotions, induced through loving-kindness meditation, build consequential personal resources. Journal of Personality and Social Psychology, 2008. 95 (5): p. 1045-1062.

19. Neff, K. and R. Vonk, Self-compassion versus global self-esteem: Two different ways of relating to oneself. Journal of Personality, 2009. 77: p. 23-50.

20. Krasner, M.S., et al., Association of an Educational Program in Mindful Communication With Burnout, Empathy, and Attitudes Among Primary Care Physicians. JAMA: The Journal of the American Medical Association, 2009. 302(12): p. 1284-1293.

21. Kearney, M.K., et al., Self-care of Physicians Caring for Patients at the End of Life. JAMA: The Journal of the American Medical Association, 2009. 301(11): p. 1155-1164.

22. Harrison RL, W.M., Preventing vicarious traumatization of mental health therapists: Identifying protective practices. Psychotherapy: Theory, Research, Practice, Training, 2009. 46(2)(June 2009): p. 203-219.

23. Beeson, S., Practicing Excellence - A Physician's Manual to Exceptional Healthcare. 2006, Gulf Breeze, Florida: Fire Starter Publishing.

24. Krischke, M., Hourly Rounds Reduce Rate of Patient Falls and Bedsores. NurseZone.com, 2009.

25. Garland, E.L., et al., Upward spirals of positive emotions counter downward spirals of negativity: Insights from the broaden-and-build theory and affective neuroscience on the treatment of emotion dysfunctions and deficits in psychopathology. Clinical Psychology Review, 2010. 30(7): p. 849-864.

Chapter 2 Notes

1. Youngson, R., Compassion in Healthcare - The missing dimension of healthcare reform?, 2008, NHS Confederation.

2. Kahn, M.W., Etiquette-Based Medicine. New England Journal of Medicine, 2008. 358(19): p. 1988-1989.

3. Drenkard, K.N., Integrating Human Caring Science into a Professional Nursing Practice Model. Critical Care Nursing Clinics of North America, 2008. 20(4): p. 403-414.

4. Frank, M.E.P., Physiologic effects of the smile. Direction in Psychiatry, 1996. 16(25): p. 1-8.

5. Rosenberg, E.L., et al., Linkages Between Facial Expressions of Anger and Transient Myocardial Ischemia in Men With Coronary Artery Disease. Emotion, 2001. 1(2): p. 107-115.

6. Seligman, M.E.P., Positive Health. Applied Psychology: An International ReviewN, 2008. 57: p. 3-18.

7. Quirk, M., et al., How patients perceive a doctor's caring attitude. Patient Education and Counseling, 2008. 72(3): p. 359-366.

8. Hemmerdinger, J., S. Stoddart, and R. Lilford, A systematic review of tests of empathy in medicine. BMC Medical Education, 2007. 7(1): p. 1-8.

9. Mercer, S.W., et al., The consultation and relational empathy (CARE) measure: development and preliminary validation and reliability of an empathy-based consultation process measure. Family Practice, 2004. 21(6): p. 699-705.

10. Garden, R., Expanding Clinical Empathy: An Activist Perspective. Journal of General Internal Medicine, 2009. 24(1): p. 122-125.

11. Goetz, J., D. Keltner, and E. Simon-Thomas, Compassion: An Evolutionary analysis and empirical review. Psychological Bulletin, 2010. 136(3): p. 351-74.

12. Janssen, A.L. and R.D. MacLeod, What does care mean? Perceptions of people approaching the end of life. Palliative & Supportive Care, 2010. 8(04): p. 433-440.

13. Larson, E.B. and X. Yao, Clinical Empathy as Emotional Labor in the Patient-Physician Relationship. JAMA: The Journal of the American Medical Association, 2005. 293(9): p. 1100-1106.

Chapter 3 Notes

1. Galvin, K.T. and L. Todres, Embodying Nursing Openheartedness. Journal of Holistic Nursing, 2009. 27(2): p. 141-149.

2. Maben, J., S. Latter, and J.M. Clark, The sustainability of ideals, values and the nursing mandate: evidence from a longitudinal qualitative study. Nursing Inquiry, 2007. 14(2): p. 99-113.

3. Youngson, R., Taking off the armor. Illness, Crisis and Loss, 2010. 18(Number 1): p. 79-82.

4. Waitemata District Health Board, Report into the Operating Theatre Fire Accident, Waitakere Hospital, 17th August, 2002, Medsafe, New Zealand.

5. Bismark, M.M., The power of apology. The New Zealand medical journal, 2009. 122(1304): p. 96-106.

6. Medically Induced Trauma Support Services. Available from: http://www.mitts.org.

7. Rowe, M., Doctors' responses to medical errors. Critical Reviews in Oncology/ Hematology, 2004. 52(3): p. 147-163.

8. Rowe, M., The Rest Is Silence. Health Affairs, 2002. 21(4): p. 232-236.

9. Remen, R.N., In the service of life. Noetic Sciences Review, 1996. 37(Spring 1996): p. 24.

10. Neff, K., The role of self-compassion in development: A healthier way to relate to oneself. Human Development, 2009. 52: p. 211-214.

11. Brown, S.D., M.J. Goske, and C.M. Johnson, Beyond substance abuse: stress, burnout, and depression as causes of physician impairment and disruptive behavior. Journal of the American College of Radiology : JACR, 2009. 6(7): p. 479-85.

12. Neff, K. and R. Vonk, Self-compassion versus global self-esteem: Two different ways of relating to oneself. Journal of Personality, 2009. 77: p. 23-50.

13. Quest for Life. Available from: http://www.questforlife.com.au.

14. Heider, J., The Tao of leadership. 1986, Aldershot: Wildwood House.

Chapter 4 Notes

1. Seligman, M.E.P., Learned optimism. 1990, New York, N.Y.: Pocket Books. 319 p.

2. Gilbert, P., et al., Self-Criticism and Self-Warmth: An Imagery Study Exploring Their Relation to Depression. Journal of Cognitive Psychotherapy, 2006. 20: p. 183-200.

3. Gilbert, P., Introducing compassion-focused therapy. Adv Psychiatr Treat, 2009. 15(3): p. 199-208.

4. Garland, E.L., et al., Upward spirals of positive emotions counter downward spirals of negativity: Insights from the broaden-and-build theory and affective neuroscience on the treatment of emotion dysfunctions and deficits in psychopathology. Clinical Psychology Review, 2010. 30(7): p. 849-864.

5. Gilbert, P. and S. Procter, Compassionate mind training for people with high shame and self-criticism: overview and pilot study of a group therapy approach. Clinical Psychology & Psychotherapy, 2006. 13(6): p. 353-379.

6. Krasner, M.S., et al., Association of an Educational Program in Mindful Communication With Burnout, Empathy, and Attitudes Among Primary Care Physicians. JAMA: The Journal of the American Medical Association, 2009. 302(12): p. 1284-1293.

7. Shapiro, S.L., et al., Mindfulness-Based Stress Reduction for health care professionals: Results from a randomized trial. International Journal of Stress Management, 2005. 12, : p. 164-176.

8. Siegel, R.D., C.K. Germer, and A. Olendzki, Mindfulness: What is it? Where did It come from?, in Clinical Handbook of Mindfulness., F. Didonna, Editor 2008, Springer: New York. p. 2-24.

9. Ludwig, D.S. and J. Kabat-Zinn, Mindfulness in Medicine. JAMA: The Journal of the American Medical Association, 2008. 300(11).

10. Weibel, D.T., A loving-kindness intervention: Boosting compassion for self and others, 2007, ProQuest Psychology Journals.

11. Shapiro, S. and S. Izett, Meditation: A universal tool for cultivating empathy, in Mindfulness and the therapeutic relationship., S. Hick and T. Bien, Editors. 2008, Guilford Press: New York. p. 161-175.

12. Epstein, R., MIndful practice JAMA: The Journal of the American Medical Association, 1999. 282(9): p. 833-839.

Chapter 5 Notes

1. Giltay, E.J., et al., Dispositional optimism and all-cause and cardiovascular mortality in a prospective cohort of elderly dutch men and women. Archives of general psychiatry, 2004. 61(11): p. 1126-35.

2. Buchanan, G.M., Explanatory style and coronary heart disease., in Explanatory style, G. Buchanan and M. Seligman, Editors. 1995, Erlbaum: Hillsdale, NJ. p. 225-232.

3. Veenhoven, R., Healthy happiness: effects of happiness on physical health and the consequences for preventive health care. Journal of Happiness Studies, 2008. 9(3): p. 449-469.

4. Seligman, M.E.P., Positive Health. Applied Psychology: An International ReviewN, 2008. 57: p. 3-18.

5. Rosenberg, E.L., et al., Linkages Between Facial Expressions of Anger and Transient Myocardial Ischemia in Men With Coronary Artery Disease. Emotion, 2001. 1(2): p. 107-115.

6. Szeto, A., et al., Oxytocin attenuates NADPH-dependent superoxide activity and IL-6 secretion in macrophages and vascular cells. American journal of physiology. Endocrinology and metabolism, 2008. 295(6): p. E1495-501.

7. Kraus, S. and S. Sears, Measuring the Immeasurables: Development and Initial Validation of the Self-Other Four Immeasurables (SOFI) Scale Based on Buddhist Teachings on Loving Kindness, Compassion, Joy, and Equanimity. Social Indicators Research, 2009. 92(1): p. 169-181.

8. Neff, K., Self-compassion: An alternative conceptualization of a healthy attitude toward oneself. Self and Identity, 2003. 2: p. 85-102.

9. Allen, A.B. and M.R. Leary, Self-Compassion, Stress, and Coping. Social and personality psychology compass, 2010. 4(2): p. 107-118.

10. Pace, T.W.W., et al., Effect of compassion meditation on neuroendocrine, innate immune and behavioral responses to psychosocial stress. Psychoneuroendocrinology,, 2009. 34: p. 87-98.

11. Rockliff, H., et al., A pilot exploration of heart rate variability and salivary cortisol responses to compassion-focused imagery. Clinical Neuropsychiatry, 2008. 5(3): p. 135-139.

12. Davidson, R.J., et al., Alterations in Brain and Immune Function Produced by Mindfulness Meditation. Psychosom Med, 2003. 65(4): p. 564-570.

13. Cohen, S., et al., Positive emotional style predicts resistance to illness after experimental exposure to rhinovirus or influenza a virus. Psychosomatic medicine, 2006. 68(6): p. 809-15.

14. Lipton, B.H., The biology of belief : unleashing the power of consciousness, matter & miracles. 2008, London: Hay House.

15. Gould, K.L., et al., Improved stenosis geometry by quantitative coronary arteriography after vigorous risk factor modification. The American journal of cardiology, 1992. 69(9): p. 845-53.

16. Ornish, D., Avoiding revascularization with lifestyle changes: The Multicenter Lifestyle Demonstration Project. The American journal of cardiology, 1998. 82(10B): p. 72T-76T.

17. Ornish, D., et al., Changes in prostate gene expression in men undergoing an intensive nutrition and lifestyle intervention. Proceedings of the National Academy of Sciences of the United States of America, 2008. 105(24): p. 8369-74.

18. Ornish, D., et al., Intensive lifestyle changes may affect the progression of prostate cancer. The Journal of urology, 2005. 174(3): p. 1065-9; discussion 1069-70.

19. Ornish, D., et al., Increased telomerase activity and comprehensive lifestyle changes: a pilot study. The lancet oncology, 2008. 9(11): p. 1048-57.

20. Firth-Cozens, J., Interventions to improve physicians' well-being and patient care. Social Science & Medicine, 2001. 52(2): p. 215-222.

21. Howard, F., Managing stress or enhancing wellbeing? Positive psychology's contributions to clinical supervision. Australian Psychologist, 2008. 43(2): p. 105-113.

22. Bogue, R.J., et al., Secrets of Physician Satisfaction: Study identifies pressure points and reveals life practices of highly satisfied doctors. The Physician Executive, 2006: p. 30-34.

23. Adler, M.G., The Sociophysiology of Caring in the Doctor-patient Relationship. Journal of General Internal Medicine, 2002. 17: p. 883-890.

24. Hojat, M., et al., Patient perceptions of physician empathy, satisfaction with physician, interpersonal trust, and compliance. Int J Med Educ, 2010. 1: p. 83-87.

25. Geller, G., et al., What do clinicians derive from partnering with their patients?: A reliable and valid measure of "personal meaning in patient care". Patient Education and Counseling, 2008. 72(2): p. 293-300.

26. Shanafelt, T.D., Enhancing Meaning in Work. JAMA: The Journal of the American Medical Association, 2009. 302(12): p. 1338-1340.

27. Krasner, M.S., et al., Association of an Educational Program in Mindful Communication With Burnout, Empathy, and Attitudes Among Primary Care Physicians. JAMA: The Journal of the American Medical Association, 2009. 302(12): p. 1284-1293.

28. Moerman, D.E. and W.B. Jonas, Deconstructing the Placebo Effect and Finding the Meaning Response. Annals of Internal Medicine, 2002. 136(6): p. 471-476.

Chapter 6 Notes

1. Brewin, C.R., Understanding cognitive behaviour therapy: A retrieval competition account. Behaviour Research and Therapy, 2006. 44(6): p. 765-784.

2. Adler, M.G. and N.S. Fagley, Appreciation: Individual Differences in Finding Value and Meaning as a Unique Predictor of Subjective Well-Being. Journal of Personality, 2005. 73(1): p. 79-114.

3. Doidge, N., The brain that changes itself : stories of personal triumph from the frontiers of brain science. 2008, London: Penguin Books.

Chapter 7 Notes

1. Janssen, A.L. and R.D. MacLeod, What does care mean? Perceptions of people approaching the end of life. Palliative & Supportive Care, 2010. 8(04): p. 433-440.

2. Kolcaba, K. and M. DiMarco, Comfort theory and its application to pediatric nursing Pedocatric Nursing, 2005. 31(3): p. 187-194.

3. Fredriksson, L., Modes of relating in a caring conversation: a research synthesis on presence, touch and listening. Journal of Advanced Nursing, 1999. 30(5): p. 1167-76.

4. Coakley, A.B. and M.E. Duffy, The effect of therapeutic touch on postoperative patients. Journal of holistic nursing : official journal of the American Holistic Nurses' Association, 2010. 28(3): p. 193-200.

5. Whitley, J.A. and B.L. Rich, A double-blind randomized controlled pilot trial examining the safety and efficacy of therapeutic touch in premature infants. Advances in neonatal care : official journal of the National Association of Neonatal Nurses, 2008. 8(6): p. 315-33.

6. Dominguez Rosales, R., et al., Effectiveness of the application of therapeutic touch on weight, complications, and length of hospital stay in preterm newborns attended in a neonatal unit. Enfermeria clinica, 2009. 19(1): p. 11-5.

7. Monroe, C.M., The effects of therapeutic touch on pain. Journal of holistic nursing : official journal of the American Holistic Nurses' Association, 2009. 27(2): p. 85-92.

8. Aghabati, N., E. Mohammadi, and Z. Pour Esmaiel, The effect of therapeutic touch on pain and fatigue of cancer patients undergoing chemotherapy. Evidence-based complementary and alternative medicine : eCAM, 2010. 7(3): p. 375-81.

9. Larden, C.N., M.L. Palmer, and P. Janssen, Efficacy of therapeutic touch in treating pregnant inpatients who have a chemical dependency. Journal of holistic nursing : official journal of the American Holistic Nurses' Association, 2004. 22(4): p. 320-32.

10. Woods, D.L., C. Beck, and K. Sinha, The effect of therapeutic touch on behavioral symptoms and cortisol in persons with dementia. Forschende Komplementarmedizin, 2009. 16(3): p. 181-9.

11. Movaffaghi, Z., et al., Effects of therapeutic touch on blood hemoglobin and hematocrit level. Journal of holistic nursing : official journal of the American Holistic Nurses' Association, 2006. 24(1): p. 41-8.

12. Marta, I.E., et al., The effectiveness of therapeutic touch on pain, depression and sleep in patients with chronic pain: clinical trial. Revista da Escola de Enfermagem da U S P, 2010. 44(4): p. 1100-6.

13. Post-White, J., et al., Therapeutic massage and healing touch improve symptoms in cancer. Integrative cancer therapies, 2003. 2(4): p. 332-44.

14. Gronowicz, G.A., et al., Therapeutic touch stimulates the proliferation of human cells in culture. Journal of alternative and complementary medicine, 2008. 14(3): p. 233-9.

15. Jhaveri, A., et al., Therapeutic touch affects DNA synthesis and mineralization of human osteoblasts in culture. Journal of orthopaedic research : official publication of the Orthopaedic Research Society, 2008. 26(11): p. 1541-6.

16. Monzillo, E. and G. Gronowicz, New insights on therapeutic touch: a discussion of experimental methodology and design that resulted in significant effects on normal human cells and osteosarcoma. Explore, 2011. 7(1): p. 44-51.

17. McCraty, R., M. Atkinson, and D. Tomasino, Science of the Heart. Exploring the role of the heart in human performance, 2001, Institute of Heartmath: Bolder Creek, CA.

18. Remen, R.N., Kitchen table wisdom : stories that heal. 1996, New York: Riverhead Books. xxx, 336 p.

Chapter 8 Notes

1. Cattaneo, L. and G. Rizzolatti, The mirror-neuron system Annual Review of Neuroscience, 2004. 27(1): p. 169-192.

2. Bastiaansen, J.A., M. Thioux, and C. Keysers, Evidence for mirror systems in emotions. Philosophical transactions of the Royal Society of London. Series B, Biological sciences, 2009. 364(1528): p. 2391-404.

3. Adler, M.G., The Sociophysiology of Caring in the Doctor-patient Relationship. Journal of General Internal Medicine, 2002. 17: p. 883-890.

4. Siegel, D.J., Mindsight : the new science of personal transformation. 1st ed. 2010, New York: Bantam Books. xviii, 314 p.

5. Decety, J., The Neurodevelopment of Empathy in Humans. Developmental Neuroscience, 2010. 32(4): p. 257-267.

6. Rein, G., M. Atkinson, and R. McCraty, The physiological and psychological effects of compassion and anger. Journal for the Advancement of Medicine., 1995. 8: p. 87-105.

7. Goetz, J., D. Keltner, and E. Simon-Thomas, Compassion: An Evolutionary analysis and empirical review. Psychological Bulletin, 2010. 136(3): p. 351-74.

8. Davidson, R., Asymmetric brain function, affective style, and psychopathology: The role of early experience and plasticity. Development and Psychopathology, 1994. 6: p. 741-758.

9. Garland, E.L., et al., Upward spirals of positive emotions counter downward spirals of negativity: Insights from the broaden-and-build theory and affective neuroscience on the treatment of emotion dysfunctions and deficits in psychopathology. Clinical Psychology Review, 2010. 30(7): p. 849-864.

10. Davidson, R.J., et al., Alterations in Brain and Immune Function Produced by Mindfulness Meditation. Psychosom Med, 2003. 65(4): p. 564-570.

11. Lutz, A., et al., Regulation of the neural circuitry of emotion by compassion meditation: effects of meditative expertise. PLoS One, 2008. 3(3): p. e1897.

12. Lutz, A., et al., Long-term meditators self-induce high-amplitude gamma synchrony during mental practice. Proceedings of the National Academy of Sciences of the United States of America, 2004. 101(46): p. 16369-16373.

13. Birnie, K., M. Speca, and L.E. Carlson, Exploring self-compassion and empathy in the context of mindfulness-based stress reduction (MBSR). Stress and Health, 2010. 26(5): p. 359-371.

14. Longe, O., et al., Having a word with yourself: Neural correlates of self-criticism and self-reassurance. Neuroimage, 2010. 49(2): p. 1849-1856.

15. Farb, N., et al., Minding one's emotions: Mindfulness training alters the neural expression of sadness. Emotion, 2010. 10(1): p. 25-33.

16. Goleman, D. and Dalai Lama XIV, Destructive emotions : and how we can overcome them : a dialogue with the Dalai Lama. 2003, London: Bloomsbury. xxiii, 404 p.

17. Bar-On, R., et al., Exploring the neurological substrate of emotional and social intelligence. Brain, 2003. 126(8): p. 1790-1800.

Chapter 9 Notes

1. Merritt Hawkins & Associates, The Physicians' Perspective:Medical Practice in 2008, The Physicians' Foundation: USA.

2. Maben, J., S. Latter, and J.M. Clark, The sustainability of ideals, values and the nursing mandate: evidence from a longitudinal qualitative study. Nursing Inquiry, 2007. 14(2): p. 99-113.

3. Zuger, A., Dissatisfaction with Medical Practice. New England Journal of Medicine, 2004. 350(1): p. 69-75.

4. Pedersen, R., Empirical research on empathy in medicine—A critical review. Patient Education and Counseling, 2009. 76 p. 307–322.

5. Wilson, G., Implementation of Releasing Time to Care - the productive ward. Journal of nursing management, 2009. 17(5): p. 647-54.

6. NHS Scotland, Releasing time to care - Evaluation, 2010.

7. Levinson, W., R. Gorawara-Bhat, and J. Lamb, A study of patient clues and physician responses in primary care and surgical settings. JAMA : the journal of the American Medical Association, 2000. 284(8): p. 1021-7.

8. Meade, C.M., A.L. Bursell, and L. Ketelsen, Effects of nursing rounds: on patients' call light use, satisfaction, and safety. The American journal of nursing, 2006. 106(9): p. 58-70.

9. Clown Doctors - The Humour Foundation. Available from: http://clowndoctors.org.au/home.html.

10. Spritzer, P., Humour can begin to reverse dementia. Personal communication 2011.

11. Takeda, M., et al., Laughter and humor as complementary and alternative medicines for dementia patients. BMC complementary and alternative medicine, 2010. 10: p. 28.

12. Gesundheit Institute. Available from: http://www.patchadams.org/.

13. Drenkard, K.N., Integrating Human Caring Science into a Professional Nursing Practice Model. Critical Care Nursing Clinics of North America, 2008. 20(4): p. 403-414.

Chapter 10 Notes

1. Senge, P. Society of Organizational Learning (SoL). Available from: http://www.solonline.org/aboutsol/who/Senge/.

2. Tiritiri Matangi Island Scientific Reserve. Available from: http://www.tiritirimatangi. org.nz.

3. Quine, L., Workplace bullying in nurses. Journal of health psychology, 2001. 6(1): p. 73-84.

4. Scott, J., C. Blanshard, and S. Child, Workplace bullying of junior doctors: cross-sectional questionnaire survey. The New Zealand medical journal, 2008. 121(1282): p. 10-4.

5. Steadman, L., et al., Experience of workplace bullying behaviours in postgraduate hospital dentists: questionnaire survey. British dental journal, 2009. 207(8): p. 379-80.

6. Hogh, A., H. Hoel, and I.G. Carneiro, Bullying and employee turnover among healthcare workers: a three-wave prospective study. Journal of nursing management, 2011. 19(6): p. 742-51.

7. Porto, G. and R. Lauve, Disruptive Clinician Behavior: A Persistent Threat to Patient Safety. Patient Safety & Quality Health Care, 2006.

8. Rosenstein, A.H. and M. O'Daniel, Disruptive behavior and clinical outcomes: perceptions of nurses and physicians. The American journal of nursing, 2005. 105(1): p. 54-64; quiz 64-5.

9. Rosenstein, A.H., H. Russell, and R. Lauve, Disruptive physician behavior contributes to nursing shortage. Study links bad behavior by doctors to nurses leaving the profession. Physician executive, 2002. 28(6): p. 8-11.

10. May, N., et al., Appreciative Inquiry in Healthcare. Positive Questions to Bring Out the Best. 2010, Brunswick, Ohio: Crown Custom Publishing, Inc.

11. Cummings, G.G., et al., Leadership styles and outcome patterns for the nursing workforce and work environment: A systematic review. International Journal of Nursing Studies, 2010. 47(3): p. 363-385.

12. Boan, D. and F. Funderburk, Healthcare Quality Improvement and Organizational Culture, 2003, Delmarve Foundation.

13. Stordeur, S., W. D'Hoore, and N.-S.G. the, Organizational configuration of hospitals succeeding in attracting and retaining nurses. Journal of Advanced Nursing, 2007. 57(1): p. 45-58.

14. PriceWaterHouseCoopers, Building the case for wellness, 2008, Heath Work Wellbeing Executive.

15. Shirely, M., Authentic Leaders Creating Healthy Work Environments for Nursing Practice. American Journal of Critical Care, 2006. 15: p. 256-267.

16. United Nations Statistics Division. Social Indicators - Indicators on Health. 2011; Available from: http://unstats.un.org/unsd/demographic/products/socind/health. htm.

17. Kelm, B., What Cuba Can Teach Us about Healthcare, in Wired 2010.

18. Bornstein, D., If the World is to be Put in Order. Vera Cordeiro, Brazil: Reforming Healthcare, in How to Change the World. Social Entrepreneurs and the Power of New Ideas2007, OUP: Oxford. p. 130-150.

19. Todres, L., K.T. Galvin, and I. Holloway, The humanization of healthcare: A value framework for qualitative research. International Journal of Qualitative Studies on Health and Well-being, 2009. 4: p. 68-77.

20. Bate, P. and G. Robert, Experience-based design: from redesigning the system around the patient to co-designing services with the patient. Quality and Safety in Health Care, 2006. 15(5): p. 307-310.

21. Dewar, B., et al., Use of emotional touchpoints as a method of tapping into the experience of receiving compassionate care in a hospital setting. Journal of Research in Nursing, 2010. 15(1): p. 29-41.

22. Dewar, B. and R. Mackay, Appreciating and developing compassionate care in an acute hospital setting caring for older people. International Journal of Older People Nursing, 2010: p. 229-308.

23. The Schwartz Center for Compassionate Healthcare. Available from: http://www.theschwartzcenter.org.

24. Lown, B.A. and C.F. Manning, The Schwartz Center Rounds: Evaluation of an Interdisciplinary Approach to Enhancing Patient-Centered Communication, Teamwork, and Provider Support. Academic Medicine, 2010. 85(6): p. 1073-1081.

25. The Kings Fund. Point of Care Programme. [cited 2011]; Available from: http://www.kingsfund.org.uk/current_projects/point_of_care/.

26. Morrison, R.S., et al., Cost Savings Associated With US Hospital Palliative Care Consultation Programs. Arch Intern Med, 2008. 168(16): p. 1783-1790.

27. Temel, J.S., et al., Early palliative care for patients with metastatic non-small-cell lung cancer. The New England Journal of Medicine, 2010. 363(8): p. 733-42.

Chapter 11 Notes

1. Youngson, R., T. Wimbrow, and T. Stacey, A crisis in maternity services: the courage to be wrong. Quality & Safety in Health Care, 2003. 12(6): p. 398-400.

2. De Bono, E., Six thinking hats. Rev. ed. 2000, London: Penguin. 192p.

3. Dewar, B. and R. Mackay, Appreciating and developing compassionate care in an acute hospital setting caring for older people. International Journal of Older People Nursing, 2010: p. 229-308.

4. May, N., et al., Appreciative Inquiry in Healthcare. Positive Questions to Bring Out the Best. 2100, Brunswick, Ohio: Crown Custom Publishing, Inc.

5. Fredrickson, B., Positivity : groundbreaking research to release your inner optimist and thrive. 2010, Richmond: Oneworld. 277 p.

6. The Schwartz Center for Compassionate Healthcare. Available from: http://www.theschwartzcenter.org.

7. Lown, B.A. and C.F. Manning, The Schwartz Center Rounds: Evaluation of an Interdisciplinary Approach to Enhancing Patient-Centered Communication, Teamwork, and Provider Support. Academic Medicine, 2010. 85(6): p. 1073-1081.

8. Wheatley, M.J., Finding our way : leadership for an uncertain time. 2005, San Francisco, Calif.: Berrett-Koehler. 300 p.

9. Jaworski, J., Synchronicity: The Inner Path of Leadership. 1996, San Francisco: Berrett-Koehler Publishers.

10. Micalizzi, D. The Task Force for Global Health: Justin's Hope Project. Available from: http://www.taskforce.org/our-work/projects/justins-hope.

Chapter 12 Notes

1. Ariely, D., Predictably irrational : the hidden forces that shape our decisions. 1st ed. 2008, New York, NY: Harper. xxii, 280 p.

2. Gladwell, M., The tipping point : how little things can make a big difference. 1st Back Bay pbk. Ed. 2002, Boston: Back Bay Books/Little, Brown. xii, 301 p.

3. Otake, K., et al., Happy people become happier through kindness: a counting kindness intervention. Journal of Happiness Studies, 2006. 7: p. 361-375.

4. Hutcherson, C., E. Seppala, and J. Gross, Loving-kindness meditation increases social connectedness. Emotion, 2008. 8(5): p. 720-724.

5. Seligman, M.E.P., et al., Positive Psychology Progress: Empirical Validation of Interventions. . American Psychologist, 2005. Vol 60(5): p. 410-421.

6. Tucker, K., Getting the most out of life: An Examination of Appreciation, Targets of Appreciation, and Sensitivity to Reward in Happier and Less Happy Individuals. Journal of Social and Clinical Psychology, 2007. 26(7): p. 791–825.

7. Polak, E. and M. McCullough, Is gratitude an alternative to materialism? Journal of Happiness Studies, 2006. 7: p. 343-360.

8. Wood, A.M., S. Joseph, and P.A. Linley, Coping style as a psychological resource of grateful people Journal of Social and Clinical Psychology, 2007. 26(9): p. 1076–1093.

9. Park, N., C. Peterson, and M.E.P. Selligman, Strengths of character and well-being. Journal of Social and Clinical Psychology, 2004. 23(5): p. 603-619.

10. Doidge, N., The brain that changes itself : stories of personal triumph from the frontiers of brain science. 2008, London: Penguin Books.

11. Garland, E.L., et al., Upward spirals of positive emotions counter downward spirals of negativity: Insights from the broaden-and-build theory and affective neuroscience on the treatment of emotion dysfunctions and deficits in psychopathology. Clinical Psychology Review, 2010. 30(7): p. 849-864.

Chapter 13 Notes

1. Wheatley, M.J., Leadership and the new science : discovering order in a chaotic world. 3rd ed. Ed. 2006, San Francisco, Calif.: Berrett-Koehler. xiv, 218 p.

2. Wheatley, M.J., Finding our way : leadership for an uncertain time. 1st ed. Ed. 2007, San Francisco, Calif.: Berrett-Koehler ; [London : McGraw-Hill, distributor]. x, 297 p.

3. Institute of Medicine, Retooling for an aging America : building the health care workforce. 2008, Washington, D.C.: National Academies Press. xvi, 300 p.

4. Wheatley, M. and D. Frieze, Leadership in the Age of Complexity: from Hero to Host, 2010: http://margaretwheatley.com/writing.html.

5. Wheatley, M. and D. Frieze, Using Emergence to Take Social Innovation to Scale, 2008, Berkana Institute: http://margaretwheatley.com/writing.html.

6. Rabow, M., J. Wrubel, and R. Remen, Authentic Community as an Educational Strategy for Advancing Professionalism: A National Evaluation of the Healer's Art Course. Journal of General Internal Medicine, 2007. 22(10): p. 1422-1428.

7. Rufsvold, R.M. and R.N. Remen, Finding Meaning in Medicine:Reclaiming the Soul of Practice. San Francisco Medicine, 2002: p. 28-30.

8. Lown, B., Prescription for survival : a doctor's journey to end nuclear madness. 1st ed. Ed. 2008, San Francisco, Calif.: Berrett-Koehler Publishers. xi, 436 p., [8] p. of plates.

SUGGESTED BOOKS AND RESOURCES

Free on-line meditation resources

- Open Your Heart
  www.open-your-heart.org.uk/index.do
- CALM Computer Assisted Learning for the mind
  www.calm.auckland.ac.nz/
- Meditation Society of Australia
  www.meditation.org.au
- Fragrant Heart – Heart Centred Meditations
  www.fragrantheart.com/
- Buddhanet – Buddha Dharma Education Association
  www.buddhanet.net/audio-meditation.htm

Recommended books

The Power of Appreciative Inquiry A Practical Guide to Positive Change. Diana Whitney & Amanda Trosten-Bloom. A comprehensive and highly practical introduction to Appreciative Inquiry, written by two of the leading practitioners.

Appreciative Inquiry in Healthcare Positive Questions to Bring Out the Best. Natalie May, Daniel Becker et al. The first major application of Appreciative Inquiry to healthcare does indeed bring out the best. This book is inspiring.

The Compassionate Mind How to use compassion to develop happiness, self-acceptance and well-being. Paul Gilbert. Written by a leading UK clinical psychologist, renowned for his work on compassionate mind therapy.

The Lost Art of Compassion Discovering the Practice of Happiness in the Meeting of Buddhism and Psychology. Lorne Ladner. This immensely helpful book explains Tibetan Buddhist concepts and practices from the perspective of Western psychology, exploring the links between compassion and happiness.

Emotional Intelligence. Daniel Goleman. A groundbreaking book that overturned the idea that IQ was the major determinant of success in life. Goleman showed that the ability to recognize emotions in oneself and others, and to manage interpersonal relationships was a crucial life skill.

Destructive Emotions And How We Can Overcome Them. A dialogue with The Dalai Lama Narrated by Daniel Goleman. A spellbinding account of the first cross-cultural dialogue between Western scientists and philosophers and The Dalai Lama.

Social Intelligence. Daniel Goleman. Building on his earlier book Emotional Intelligence, Goleman explores the latest advances in psychology and neuroscience to explore the fascinating world of interpersonal connection.

The Lost Art of Healing Practicing Compassion in Medicine. Bernard Lown. Written by a renowned cardiologist, who invented the defibrillator and developed much of modern, technological cardiology. His greatest regret, he writes, is that the introduction of technology displaced the art of healing in medical practice. An insightful and inspiring book.

Kitchen Table Wisdom Stories that Heal. Rachel Naomi Remen. This wonderful book has to be my all-time favorite as a special gift for people seeking inspiration in healthcare. Few people can read it without being profoundly moved.

Positivity Top-Notch Research Reveals the 3-to-1 Ratio That Will Change Your Life. Barbara Fredrickson. Simply the best book on the new field of positive psychology, written by one of the leading researchers.

The Brain That Changes Itself Stories of personal triumph from the frontiers of brain science. Norman Doidge. Astonishing accounts of neuroplasticity – the capacity of the human brain to heal itself from what was long thought to be irreversible damage. Among other revelations is the fact that our thoughts can switch genes on and off, altering our brain anatomy.

Mindsight The New Science of Personal Transformation. Daniel Siegel. A fascinating exploration of the interface between mind, brain and relationships and how we can achieve optimal well-being by using our capacity for attention to change the structure and function of our brains.

Leadership and the New Science Discovering order in a Chaotic World. Margaret Wheatley. A best-selling and highly acclaimed book on the realities of leading in times of turbulence and chaos, using the power of non-linear networks and self-organizing systems.

QBQ The Question Behind the Question What to Really Ask Yourself - Practicing Personal Accountability in Business and in Life. John Miller. This deceptively simple and inspiring book tells us how we can become so much more effective, and happier, by asking better questions and discovering the joy of personal accountability.

INDEX

CPSIA information can be obtained at www.ICGtesting.com
Printed in the USA
LVOW071451070113

314705LV00019B/820/P